Ketosis

Ketogenic Diet: Ketogenic Bootcamp:

The Wicked Good Ketogenic Diet Cookbook

Table of Content

Introduction..1

What is the Ketogenic Diet and Ketosis?...................4

Guidance into the fundamentals of the ketogenic diet, advice for living the keto-lifestyle..12

Ketogenic diet plan – the food you should be eating..27

A Side Effect of Ketosis..................................43

Less positive side-effects................................49

Tips for Success with Keto Diet..........................55

What to Avoid on the Ketogenic Diet?.....................58

How to Reach a State of Ketosis?.........................61

Improved cholesterol readings............................65

Reduction in blood sugar and blood pressure.............69

Other Benefits of a Ketogenic Diet.......................72

Keto-lifestyle and a complete two-week meal plan.75

Ketogenic Diet as a Permanent Lifestyle Change..114

How fast can you lose weight?...........................119

Body mass index...125

Super foods...129

Water for Weight Loss...................................139

Exercise..147

Positivity	159
Eating Out	170
Planning	176
Conclusion	178

Introduction

Do you feel tired? Unmotivated? Unable to concentrate? Do you want to lose weight and become healthier? Do you lack inspiration for healthy meal you can prepare? Are you fed up of diets costing you the earth and producing little in the way of results? If so, this book is for you. It will tell you all you need to know about a ketogenic diet, and the many benefits that this diet can have for your health. Ketogenic diets are grounded in logical science, there are specific reasons why this type of diet helps you to lose weight and burns fat, once your body enters ketosis.

Inside the book you'll learn all about foods that you can and can't eat on a Ketogenic diet. You'll learn how to reach a state of ketosis, and how you can test for this.

This book explains the improvements that will take place regarding your cholesterol; your blood sugar, and blood pressure, as well as many other benefits of a Ketogenic diet for those with epilepsy, acne, polycystic ovary syndrome (PCOS); Alzheimer's and Parkinson's.

This book has recipes that just require 5 main ingredients. There's nothing complicated about that, no specialist equipment that you need to purchase. The recipes use good wholesome food, and shows how you can make tasty and delicious food to enjoy. This book will give you lots of ideas of things to make, using simple ingredients. It will spice up meal-times and help you to stick at your diet. This diet is very affordable; by eating good wholesome food and cutting out processed carbohydrates, you'll save money, and feel full, and be healthy too.

By eating a Ketogenic diet you will:

- Have far more energy
- Be able to think clearly
- Lose excess body weight
- Control the carbohydrates you eat

Inside this book, you'll find:

- All you need to know about following a ketogenic diet
- Lots of detailed information about ketosis and your body
- Information about cholesterol and fat, which has been popularly misunderstood by many, including the medical profession.
- Many Ketogenic recipes, including some that use just 5 main ingredients, or less.

Some of the recipes you'll find in this book include:

• A delicious hearty traditional satisfying rustic Meat Pie
• Light and flavoursome breakfast muffins
• Chocolate pots
• A tasty snack of ham and cheese pockets, which is easy to rustle up in around 20 minutes.
• A low carb pizza
• Mediterranean pork chops
• Paneer curry
• Bacon wrapped and cheese stuffed burgers

Good luck with your Ketogenic diet, by following this book, and he recipes within it, you'll start to see some amazing results and be healthier than ever. The food you can eat is amazing and delicious, and will change you metabolic state, so that your body burns fat, instead of sugary carbohydrates, putting you at far less risk of diseases.

What is the Ketogenic Diet and Ketosis?

A Ketogenic diet is a diet that is low in carbohydrates. You may hear a Ketogenic diet referred to as 'Keto' for short. You may hear carbohydrates, referred to as 'carb/s' for short. More accurately the diet is high fat, medium protein and low carbohydrate.

The general definition of the word "Keto" is derived from a bodily metabolic process known as "Ketosis." This process is what allows to body to lose weight so fast while under a Ketogenic Diet.

Ketosis is also known as 'nutritional ketosis,' is essentially how many ketones you have in your blood.

What is Ketosis you say? Well, it is the process through which the body releases a chemical called Ketones which significantly helps to lower down the level of fats in our body and sustain all your activities well. When there is scarcity of carbohydrate from the food you take, the fat in your body is burnt to provide that energy, which your carbohydrate could not provide. As a consequence of the process, ketones are produced.

By following this diet you'll burn fat more quickly. This will help you to lose weight. There are other diets out there which place an emphasis on low-carbohydrates, such as the Atkins diet or LCHF (Low Carb, High Fat).

There have been many research studies that have shown that a ketogenic diet can help you to lose weight. Essentially on this diet, you'll replace carbohydrates by consuming fat instead (and whilst this may seem counterintuitive, it WILL help you to lose weight) because of the way our bodies work.

A Ketogenic diet is done with the purpose of attaining the state of ketosis. Throughout this book, you'll learn how to measure your ketone levels, and how to change your diet to reach the best ketone levels for you; ones that will help you to lose weight, and be healthy both physically and mentally.

There are at least 4 different types of Ketogenic diets that you can embark on: - but most have a figure of only eating 5% carbohydrates.

1. **A Standard Ketogenic Diet (SKD)** – Low carbohydrates, moderate protein and high fat. This diet is the one that this book mostly focusses upon. However, if you opt for any of the other ketogenic diets, this book will still be useful for them too. A Standard Ketogenic Diet typically contains: 75% fat; 20% protein and

only 5% carbohydrate – these are the KEY figures that you should keep in your mind, with every meal that you prepare for yourself, and over the course of a day.

2. **A Targeted Ketogenic Diet (TKD)** – This is for people who do a lot of exercise, and this does allow them to add more carbohydrates around their workouts. For example, if you are a person who participates in Cross-fit, you may decide to have a bowl of porridge, as a treat, after doing an early morning work-out session.

3. **High-protein Ketogenic Diet** – This is mostly the same as a standard Ketogenic diet, with the exception that you have more protein in it. So, the percentages differ, and it tends to be 60% fat; 35% protein; and still the 5% carbohydrates.

4. **Cyclical Ketogenic Diet (CKD)** – This diet tends to have 5 low carbohydrate typical ketogenic standard diet days, followed by 2 higher carbohydrate days. This diet can work well for those who work a typical Monday – Friday and find it easier to maintain a ketogenic diet at work; but may wish to relax a bit around family and friends at the weekend,

and not be so strict with carbohydrates then. This diet can work, but clearly it can take a bit longer to reach that stage of ketosis. A cyclical method can also work well for sporty people such as bodybuilders and athletes.

Eating a ketogenic diet, will help you to lose weight, and put you at less risk of disease. Research has shown that a ketogenic diet can be more effective than 'low-fat' diets. This type of diet gives you good food, that keeps you full for longer, so you don't experience many of the hunger-pang symptoms often associated with other diets. People have been found to lose more than double the amount of weight on a ketogenic diet, compared to low-fat diets. A ketogenic diet will give you more ketones, will lower your blood sugar (see Chapter 8) and improve how your body responds to insulin.

Everyone's body produces molecules known as 'ketones'. When your body is low in blood sugar, these ketones act as fuel for the body. Your body produces more ketones when you reduce how many carbohydrates you eat, and when you restrict the amount of protein you consume. This is because carbohydrates are very quickly broken down into blood sugar; and if you eat too much protein, this too turns into blood sugar.

It is the liver, which is the organ in your body, that produces ketones from fat. These ketones are then used by all of your body, including your brain, as fuel – a kind of energy!

Your body needs a lot of fuel to run efficiently. When you're on a ketogenic diet, your body starts running off the fat. Your insulin levels drop, and instead you start to burn fat. It becomes much easier for your body to tap into where you have fat stored, and start to burn this up as fuel. This will help with weight loss, but will also mean that you don't feel as hungry, and you always have energy. It certainly sounds like a win, win situation.

Your body can enter ketosis if you were to fast, and not eat anything, your body would start to burn off fat. But, clearly this would be an unhealthy way to reach ketosis. You'd probably feel quite light-headed, hungry, bad tempered and lacking in energy if you were to starve yourself. So, that is not recommended!

Instead, we recommend a ketogenic diet, whereby you eat food that will put you into a ketogenic state, but without the need to fast.

History of Ketogenic Diet

The Ketogenic Diet became very trendy as a treatment for epilepsy seizure in the mid 1920s and 30s. It was developed to give a substitute for non-mainstream fasting, which had established triumph as a therapy for epilepsy. On the other hand, the diet was ultimately discarded due to the beginning of new anticonvulsant therapies. Though it emerged that the majority cases of epilepsy could be efficiently restricted by using these medications, they were still unsuccessful to attain epileptic control in around 20% to 30% of epileptics. For these folks, and mainly children with epilepsy, the diet was re-introduced as a method for the administration of the condition.

The part of fasting in the management of the disease has been acknowledged by mankind for thousands of years and was first considered by Greek physicians and Indian physicians. An early thesis in the Hippocratic Corpus, "On the Sacred Disease," depict how a modification in diet play a role in epilepsy organization. The similar author also explains in "Epidemics" from the collection, how a man was treated for epilepsy when he desist consumption of food or drink. These days, the same diet is being considered in the medical community with applications to all sorts of diseases. Certainly, most of the medical interest in the diet is aimed to increase a line of "ketone" drugs to copy the diet. Ketones, which the body can create at some stage in fasting or "starvation," are substitute energy source for those who are insulin defiant. Insulin resistance is seen as the main cause of numerous diseases. A study shows that a diet rich in fat or low in carbohydrates and protein could preserve ketosis for a long period of time. This study also led the development of Ketogenic diet.

Normal Diet VS Ketogenic Diet

With a normal diet, the body produces insulin and glucose. Glucose is the easiest form of energy the body can convert to utilize, so it's chosen over any other energy source in the body. Insulin is created to process the glucose that's in your bloodstream. Because glucose is being used as the main source of energy, the fats you consume are not needed and are stored. Usually, on a normal diet filled with carbohydrates, the body uses glucose as its main fuel. With farming and modern agriculture, a normal diet for many people includes a diet with a large portion of calories coming from foods high in carbs such as wheat, rice, potatoes, etc.

Keto diet limits the amount of carbohydrates you consume. Minimal energy is available from glucose, and the body resorts to burning fat. The fat is converted to ketones and the ketones fuel the body. With Keto diet, ketones are the main fuel source for the body. The result is fat burning. In a state of ketosis, individuals often report being able to feel the fat burning, a steady energy flow, increased awareness, and a sharp mental focus.

Ketogenic diet draws some similarities to other low carb diets including Atkins and Paleo. These low carb diets are more similar to a hunter gatherer diet in which carb consumption was limited to carbs found in fruits and vegetables.

Guidance into the fundamentals of the ketogenic diet, advice for living the keto-lifestyle.

Good Advice for a Ketogenic Diet

1. Drink Plenty of Water

This is good advice for any diet, but it's sensible to ensure you're well hydrated. This means that your body works at its best. If you can drink 3 litres of water a day, this is a really good amount. It will help you to lose weight, your skin to be hydrated and youthful looking, and your body's organs to work correctly and to flush out any toxins. The more water you drink, the easier you'll find this to do each day. Whilst at first, you may need to make more frequent trips to the toilet, this will lessen the more the days go by and your body adjust to it.

2. Fasting

Some people on a ketogenic diet also find that fasting is beneficial. This can help you achieve the state of ketosis, because you won't be consuming calories, in terms of protein or carbohydrates. It can be sensible to do a low-carbohydrate diet for a few days before embarking on fasting, but many people find this beneficial. There's a lot of talk and diets that involve eating for 5 days, and fasting (where you only consume 600 calories per day) for two days. People lose a lot of weight on this technique, and it's also supposed to improve your memory and clarity of thought, and to stave off later life diseases such as dementia and Alzheimer's. Some people, rather than doing the 5 day eating and 2 day fasting, decide to fast a bit each day, and try to extend the time that they fast, so that once they've gone to bed, they then don't eat breakfast, but instead wait and have a late lunch, so to extend their fast. It is important to keep well hydrated when you're fasting, so keep drinking, ideally water, but other drinks (providing they're not sugary soft drinks) are fine too.

3. Eat Healthy Salt

Healthy salt, almost seems like an oxymoron, a contradiction in terms; as we're told by society so much that a lot of our food already has salt in it, and not to add it to food, and that salt is bad for you. When we eat a lot of carbohydrates, we also tend to have more insulin. But, when we cur out carbohydrates in our diets, we have less insulin, our kidneys get rid of a lot of sodium, which is why it's important for us to consume healthy salt, on a low carbohydrate diet, such as the ketogenic diet. A good healthy salt, which you can add 3-5g of per day to your diet, is pink Himalayan rock salt (this is approximately a tea-spoon throughout the course of a day, you could put a sprinkling here and there on your food). Other ways that you can get healthy salt into your system, is by consuming organic broth. You can also add ¼ tspoon to 16oz of water and drink that throughout the day. You can eat cucumber and celery which have natural sodium in them, and are also low carbohydrate. Celery in particular is very good, as you burn more calories chewing and eating it, and digesting it because of the fibre it contains, than the calories that the celery itself has. You can also eat salty sea vegetables such as kelp and nori to dishes and this will increase the good salt you have; finally, there are certain snacks you can eat, such as salted macadamia nuts an salted pumpkin seeds which are delicious as a snack, but will also give you good salt.

There is a huge difference between what we know as the white common table salt and the pink Himalayan salt. Table salt has been heated to over 1,200 degrees Fahrenheit to allegedly 'purify' it. This type of salt is 97.5% sodium chloride, and contains 2.5% of additives. Because of this process, this destroys all of the natural minerals and goodness that salt contains. There are additives in table salt, which prevent it from all clumping together. Table salt can often contain iodine, or fluoride. Whereas, pink Himalayan salt, contains 84 essential minerals that the body needs. It is 85% sodium chloride and 15% minerals. It's a really good source of magnesium, and research has shown that at least 80% of people are deficient in magnesium. By eating Himalayan pink salt, this makes the cells in your body have just the right amount of pH level. Himalayan pink salt, helps the blood sugar in your body to remain at a good level, and finally it helps you to have a good night's sleep, which always makes you feel much better, and rejuvenated and ready to take on the world.

4. Exercise

When you're on a Ketogenic diet, it's crucial that you're also participating in high intensity exercise. By doing this you'll help your body transport those glucose molecules in your blood into your liver and muscles. The more exercise you do, the more easily this process occurs. When you achieve ketosis maintaining a good exercise regime is important, because with time you'll be able to adapt to allowing some more carbohydrates in your diet. The type of exercises that are particularly effective for this type of diet include: squats, push-ups, pull ups and pull-downs and bent over rows. Many people have found that cross-fit is a particularly good exercise regime or something like circuit training. If you have lots of resistance training exercises, which include sprint running, and walking this will help you to maintain ketosis. Your exercise needn't be excessive. You could do resistance training for 20 minutes 2 days, then spend a day doing more relaxed walking; do another 2 days of resistance training, and again spend a day doing something less energetic, but still getting exercise.

5. Maintaining a healthy digestive system

Sometimes people on a Ketogenic diet can find that they suffer from constipation. There are many reasons why this could occur. It could be that the individual has some issues in their good and can have too much bad bacteria there, or candida. It could be that they're not consuming enough fibre, in the way of vegetables, food and drink. One of the key reasons is that the person is dehydrated, and simply just doesn't have enough moisture in the food, and the body tried to extract water from the food, and then the food just become stuck in the intestines and doesn't move along freely and comfortably. I can't stress enough; how important it is to try to drink around 3 litres of water a day (please see point 1 above). Your urine should be clear and not dark yellow. If your urine is dark yellow, then that's a key sign you're dehydrated (another reason could be that you have a lot of vitamin C in your body, and your body is flushing that out, but if you've not consumed vitamin C, and haven't been drinking enough, then it's a sign you're dehydrated.) A further reason for constipation is that you don't have enough electrolytes in your body, minerals, such as sodium, magnesium, calcium and potassium – this is why eating pink Himalayan rock salt can be a good idea (please see point 3 above). If you are chronically stressed, then this is another thing that can stop your intestines contracting as they should, and moving faeces along your gut. There are things you can do to prevent constipation on a Ketogenic diet, and this includes consuming products that contain good bacteria, you can eat probiotic yoghurts, you can take acidophilus tablets from a health-food shop, each fermented foods, such as sauerkraut, and coconut water. Drink lots of water, and add in Himalayan salt (just a quarter of a teaspoon) into this. If you can drink a 'green' drink a day, such as a smoothie containing apple, spinach, kiwi and kale, this will put more good minerals in your body, such as potassium, magnesium and calcium and help your digestive system greatly.

6. Monitor your protein consumption

You need to be eating the right amount of protein for your body. If you eat an excessive amount, then your body will turn it into glucose, which is what we're trying to avoid your body having too much of on a Ketogenic diet. If you're not able to maintain the state of ketosis very well, then it's certainly worth monitoring how much protein you're consuming. People will differ depending on their body type, and how much exercise they do. If you're doing a great deal of resistance training, then you may need more protein than a person who is doing aerobic exercise. As a general rule of thumb, you should be eating 1 gram of protein, for every kilogram that your body weight is. It's good to split this protein up into 2 or 3 servings over the course of the day, and not eat it all at once.

7. Select Carbohydrates carefully

A ketogenic diet, is by nature, very low carbohydrate. But, when you do consume carbohydrates, there are certain types that are better for you than others. If you can opt to have non-starchy vegetables and low-glycemic (this means that it will have a minimal effect on how much glucose circulates around your blood); fruit, such as lemons, limes, ½ Granny Smith apple in a green smoothie; or some berries in a protein shake, these are much better for you. When you come out of ketosis, you can add foods like berries, sweet potatoes, grass-fed butter, and cinnamon into your diet. On low carb days, the most you should be putting into smoothies would be ½ a Granny Smith apple, 1 carrot or 1 beetroot. Coconuts are good for you to eat, because these contain a good amount of fatty acids.

8. Use MCT Oil

MCT stands for a Medium Chain Triglyceride. Using this type of oil, will allow you to maintain ketosis, and also eat more protein and carbohydrates. A ketogenic diet means that 80-90% of the calories you consume will come from fat. If you have MCT oil, then this will reduce your fats to 60-70% because MCT oils are turned immediately into ketones, and used as fuel for the body. Coconut oil isn't MCT oil. MCT oil is 100% medium chain triglyceride whereas coconut oil is a mixture. You can use MCT oil to cook with; you can add it to protein shakes, smoothies, tea and coffee etc, and this will ensure that your ketone levels are maintained throughout the course of the day.

9. Reduce Stress

If you are suffering from chronic stress, you will not be able to achieve a state of ketosis. If something is causing chronic stress in your life, then probably your attention should be focussed upon relieving that stress, rather than focussing so much on a Ketogenic diet. This doesn't mean you have to eat a ton of carbohydrates, but you certainly don't need to be so strict or hard on yourself. Just reduce your carbohydrates a bit; sort whatever is stressing you out, and then return to the diet at a later point. When you're in a state of chronic stress, stress hormones will be raised and this in turn raises your blood sugar, to that your adrenaline is high and you're in a state of 'flight or fight'. If your level of stress continues, then your blood sugar increases, and your ketones decrease. My advice would be to work on dealing with whatever is causing the stress; there are some things in life which are out of control, but we can find the best ways of dealing with issues. Some things take more time than others, but it can vastly reduce stress, to know that you're making progress towards sorting out a problem, even if that progress is slow-going. It can be useful to get a page of A4 paper, and write down one side of it, all the things that are bothering you (issues) and making you feel stressed – try to break these down as much as possible into small chunks. Then write on the right hand side of the page, how you will resolve these issues (solutions). Most things can be overcome, or at least dealt with in a way that makes it manageable. Remember that you are a strong person; ensure that you eat as healthily as you can – if you eat lots of sugar food, this causes inflammation and makes our bodies weak, eating good food such as avocados, eggs, coconut oil, non-starchy vegetables, grass fed meat, almonds and walnuts, will make you feel better and more able to tackle any issues deftly. Definitely ensure that you drink lots of water, at least 3 litres a day, because this will help you in so many ways, physically and mentally. One really nice technique to give you a sunshine lift, is to drink lemon water. Lemon naturally gives you energy, it hydrates you, gives you oxygen, so drinking lemon water will make you feel rejuvenated, revitalized and it's very refreshing. Lemon water will boost your immune system, it will detox your system flushing out any toxins. It will make your skin have less wrinkles and blemishes. Lemon is excellent to get rid of any respiratory complains. It will help with weight loss. It will help to purify your blood and reduce infection and inflammation. Try to get out for some exercise/fresh-air/a change of scenery whenever you're able, this will help to lift your mood. Be confident that you can find solutions to all of your problems and overcome any hurdles. It can be helpful to read affirmative statements to yourself each day, and this will help you to become more confident. Use the power of visualization to imagine yourself in any situation you wish to be in. There are various herbs you can use that will help to reduce stress too: Panax Ginseng (Asian Ginseng) is used for well-being, and as an anti-depressant. Rhodiola (Golden Root) is used to reduce stress, depression and fatigue. Holy Basil is said to alleviate stress, and also to help with headaches, colds and aid the digestive system. Basil has the most amazing scent, and is so versatile for use in cooking, and smoothies/drinks.

10.   Get a good night's sleep

If you aren't sleeping well, then this will have an effect, similar to point 9 above of you being stressed. As a result your blood sugar will rise. Ensure that you go to sleep at a sensible time at night, ideally before 11pmm, and ensure that your room is suitably dark, so that you're not disturbed by street lights, or dawn light coming through the windows. It's good to try and get between 7 – 9 hours of sleep per night. If you're stressed, then you need more sleep. Ensure your room is not too hot and stuffy, ideally have a window open slightly to get a little fresh air circulating, or have air conditioning or a fan on. If you're sensitive to light or noise, then consider wearing an eye-mask or ear-plugs so that you're disrupted as little as possible.

Following these 10 points above, can help you achieve and maintain a state of Ketosis. Following the above can put your body into a state where you burn fat for body fuel and to give you the ability to think clearly and sharply, and can prevent you craving and consuming carbohydrates, and as a result feeling lethargic and cotton-wool-headed. By following the above 10 points, you'll be giving yourself the best possible head-start for your Ketogenic diet. You'll lose weight and have a leaned and toned physique and lots of energy, so that you'll able to participate fully in all aspects of life.

Is there anyone who a ketogenic diet is not Suitable for?

Most people can follow a Ketogenic diet, with the following exceptions that require you to seek medical advice first: If you're breastfeeding; If you're Diabetic; and if you have High Blood Pressure. This isn't to say that you can't start a ketogenic diet, but it is essential to check with your Dr first.

Diabetic

If you're diabetic you MUST check with your Doctor before embarking on a ketogenic diet, and heed their advice. However, a ketogenic diet, could actually be really good for your diabetes. If you have Type II diabetes, by following a ketogenic diet you could start to reduce your diabetes. If you have Type I diabetes you can increase the control that you have over your blood sugar with a ketogenic diet, which should mean you'll feel high or hypo. When you start a ketogenic diet, this may impact upon your insulin levels, and you may need to lower these. When you eat less carbohydrates, your blood sugar won't be raised as much from them, which will mean you need less insulin in order to regulate your blood sugar levels. If you continued to take the same level of insulin that you did prior to starting a ketogenic diet, then this could mean you'd end up with low blood sugar, also known as hypoglycaemia. If you decide to follow a ketogenic diet, it's important to monitor your blood sugar closely, act accordingly with insulin, and regularly be checked by a Doctor. You may need to lower your insulin by 30-50% but your Doctor will advise you on this. It's always possible to have a lower dose of insulin and top it up later, rather than by taking too much.

If you're diabetic, but at a level where you manage your diabetes with your diet, or just with Metformin, then you don't have to be so careful about monitoring and the ketogenic diet should be fine for you to adapt to.

When you eat a ketogenic diet, after a while this will result in the state known as ketosis. If you have Type 1 diabetes and have achieved ketosis, you're close to the state of ketoacidosis. If you were to forget your insulin (or something goes wrong with the device that gives you, your insulin) in this state then this could require urgent medical assistance at the hospital. Advice for people with Type 1 diabetes, is to work on just having a moderate carbohydrate diet, rather than cutting them out altogether and entering ketosis. You could also add two portions of fruit per day to your diet, if you're Type 1 diabetes.

You can recognise if you're entering ketoacidosis, if you start to experience the following symptoms: being very thirsty, feeling sick, actually being sick, and being muddled and unable to think straight. If these symptoms occur, you could try eating some carbohydrates, and be sure to get medical advice.

High Blood Pressure

Eating a very low carbohydrate diet may reduce your high blood pressure. The key caveat is that if you're on medication for high blood pressure and start this diet, your blood pressure may drop as a result of the diet and your medication combined, and therefore become too low. If you find yourself feeling lethargic, or dizzy then it can be worth checking your blood pressure (you can buy machines to check this yourself at home); or going to your Dr or chemists who will be able to check this for you. If you check your own blood pressure and find it is lower than 120/80 then you should speak to your Dr as soon as possible and discuss your blood pressure medication.

Some low carb diets can suggest that you have salty drinks such as Bovril or Bouillon in your first few weeks of a low carb diet, because this can help prevent against headaches that some people experience as a result of cutting out carbs. But if you have high blood pressure you shouldn't be drinking these. You should only have these if your blood pressure is stable. Having anything with salt in, could increase your blood pressure which clearly is not good if your blood pressure is already high! If you are on a low carb diet and experiencing headaches, these will pass once you progress into the diet, it's worth powering through them.

Types of food you can eat on a ketogenic diet?

Meat, such as bacon; pork chops/steaks; beef or lamb mince; roasted chicken; fish; shrimps; salmon; butter; cauliflower; lettuce; asparagus; avocadoes; mushrooms; broccoli; eggs; oil; cucumber; peppers; lemon; nuts; cheese; cabbage and cream.

Ketogenic diet plan – the food you should be eating

What is your health and fitness goal? Weight Loss? Cutting fat? The meal plan should be designed based on your motivation and desired outcome.

If your goal is weight loss, it's as simple as entering a state of ketosis and maintaining a calorie deficit. However, if you don't enter ketosis, or fail to maintain ketosis, weight loss goals may be compromised. You must enter ketosis, maintain that metabolic state, and in order to have successful weight loss with Keto. This means eating a diet high in fat, moderate in protein, and low in carbohydrates. For cutting fat and maintaining your weight, it's as simple as entering and maintaining ketosis and maintaining a calorie balance.

Calorie Deficit Explained

The weight loss, weight gain, and weight maintenance formulas are simple. It comes down to calorie intake vs calorie expenditure (energy needs)

Weight maintenance: Calorie intake=Calorie expenditure

Weight gain: Calorie intake>Calorie expenditure

Weight loss: Calorie intake<Calorie expenditure

Macros Explained

You hear people at the gym tossing the word back and forth like a kettlebell. Macro. Macro this, macro that. What exactly is it?

Macros stand for macronutrients. You hear people at the gym tossing the word back and forth like a kettlebell. *Macro.* Macro this, macro that. What exactly is it? Your macros are the daily intake of the three main nutrients that affect weight and your overall health, which are fats, protein, and carbohydrates. Fats have 9cals/gram, proteins and carbs have 4cals/g.

Fat = 9cals/g

Protein = 4cals/g

Carbs = 4cals/g

Fats are 90% keto, which is why they're such an efficient fuel for your body to use on a daily basis. Fats enter your body, are processed in the liver, and break down into various components your body needs to stay in top shape, such as glycerol. The remaining 10%, in case you're wondering, is a little bit of anti-keto glucose (10%) that happens when fats break down.

Carbs are completely anti-ketogenic. They break down into sugar (glucose) and consequently raise your blood sugar and your insulin levels, which translates to (unwanted) fat storage.

Proteins are approximately half-ketogenic, somewhere around 45%. The remaining percentage is broken down into glucose and raises insulin levels.

All of these macros have a different effect on how your body uses food, whether efficiently as an energy source, or for storage (fat) in case of perceived emergency. Maintaining a balance of these macros is all-important not only to the ketogenic diet, but also to overall health. Macros are metabolized (read: burned) in the furnace of our bodies, becoming the fuel that drives us through life. So we need to know about macros in order to prime that furnace (the scientific term for your furnace is 'metabolic path.' Just think of each of these macros as being a kind of highway to health.)

Macro #1: Fats.

Fats are used by your body to make repairs on damaged muscles, organs, cells, tissues, etc. You consume them, they're processed in the liver, and they circulate in the form of glycerol or other important fatty acids, acting as body repairmen.

Macro #2: Carbs.

Carbohydrates are a pre-ketogenic person's energy supply. They become glucose (sugar), which the body then uses for a boost. Unfortunately, that sugar rush releases insulin, which stockpiles glucose in the forms of both glycogen (a different kind of sugar) and fat cells. The ketogenic diet is designed to minimize carb consumption and maximize burning of glucose, glycogen, and fat. On this diet, your body is becoming far more efficient at processing.

Macro #3: Protein.

Through complex biological processes, proteins are broken down into amino acids. These amino acids break down into further compounds and become the basic building tools our body needs to repair itself after the strain of daily life (or hard workouts.) Amino acids facilitate connections between neurons in our body and brain. Ingest an overt amount of protein and it becomes stored as glucose which, as we've seen already, is sugar that the body will then rely on for energy.

Macro Counting

Counting macros is a complex task. You can get into number-crunching macros in detail on any number of free websites, which will guide you through the calculations. Keeping track of your macros is an important part of committing to a ketogenic diet, because macros are essentially what will keep you in (or out) of ketosis.

Accurately Counting Carbs

While calculating macros can get tricky, calculating net carbs is easy and will help you stay in ketosis. In unscientific terms, carbs have two parts: the part that breaks down into glucose (which you don't want), and the part that's fiber (which you do want). So when calculating carbs for their net value, subtract fiber from the total carbs. For example, if a food item has 15 carbs but 10 of them are fiber, then net carbs are only 5.

But What If ...

You suddenly stop losing weight? Not just for that erratic week or two we mentioned earlier. What if you're stuck after a month, and just not seeing any more numbers moving? First of all, remember that the numbers aren't fully reliable, so you may want to use a tape measure to check inch loss. That could be wholly different from what you're seeing on the scale, given that size loss doesn't always equal weight loss.

If it's been longer than a month and you're absolutely sure you've plateaued, don't start reducing immediately. That's right. Don't. Your body just figured out how to work with this new regime and is efficiently burning calories. If you cut back, you may confuse things all over again. Try other alternatives before you decide to revise your caloric intake. For instance, try logging your foods for a few days, to make sure extra carbs and sugar aren't sneaking in. It's easy to slip back into old habits, so you may have fallen out of the ketogenic diet without noticing. Check your macros, to make sure they're in balance. Rearrange the number of calories you eat in a given time period, so maybe you're eating the bulk of your calories in the morning and at lunch, and minimal calories for dinner, just for a few days to rev things up again. Amp up your exercise. HIIT is outstanding for building endurance, which helps your body learn to better process glucose. Be patient and you should start to see a change before long. Don't give up and go back to the habits you had before going ketogenic. This diet is proven to work. You just have to stick to it consistently and with the awareness that sometimes there will be natural stalls in the overall movement toward weight loss and health.

Using the Keto Calculator

You can make use of the keto calculator to figure out what you need to eat every day, below is an explanation of each element required to use the calculator. Estimated body fat %, estimated calorie expenditure, and desired approach to macros.

First, you're going to need to put your measurements into the calculator and your total body fat percentage. If unsure of your body fat percentage, then you can visually estimate the amount of body fat you have.

Estimating Body Fat

Body fat can be simply estimated using a body fat calculator estimator, using calipers, or estimating based on the descriptions below.

5-9% Body Fat

For men who have 5-9% body fat, muscles will show noticeably with clear definition and clear vascularity in muscles. The essential body fat for men is 2%-5%.

It is not healthy for women to have less than 10%-13% body fat.

10-14%

Men who are between 10-14% body fat will have a separation amongst muscles, but not in all muscles. The veins will mostly show on their arms and sometimes their legs.

Women are usually in this body fat range if are competitive athletes. The essential body fat for a woman is 10%-13% while it's 2%-5% for men. This is the range for bodybuilders, both women and men, are seen in, but it's not considered healthy for long-term. Muscles will be clearly distinct and divided for women, and vascularity is obvious over the entire body.

15-19%

Men who are in this range will have a lean look with less muscle visibility and vascularity. The definition of their muscles recedes and there isn't a clear separation between muscles. Most of the vascularity are gone, but some will be seen on the arms.

For women, the thighs, hips, and behind will have less shape due to a lack of body fat. Many fitness models, female athletes and bikini models are in this range because there is still a clear definition of muscles. Vascularity can be seen on the arms and legs, and there's still a separation between muscles.

20-24%

This is the average body fat range for men. The separation between the muscles groups is nonexistent, and there is not any vascularity in the muscle groups. There will be a little fat on the stomach, but it's not rounded.

For women, the separation between the muscles and the definition between the muscles is less noticeable. This is the ranges that most female athletes will fall in and it's considered very fit.

25-29%

For men, any range above 25%+ is considered obese. Men in this range usually have a little belly and there is no visible separation of muscles and vascularity.

For women, this is an average body fat percent. Curves start to form in the hips and there is more body fat around the thigh and butt.

30-34%

For men, the fat begins to distribute around the body and the waist looks larger compared to the hips. The stomach is noticeably more round and the chin fat begins to form.

For women, their fat begins to show around the thighs, hips, and butt. In the range, the thighs and behind are more rounded and pronounced.

35-39%

For men, the stomach begins to gain more and more fat around it and will be over forty inches. The stomach has a clear protrusion and hangs.

For women, the face and neck begin to gain some fat. The stomach also starts to gain fat and is protruding. Over thirty-two inches for waist size is in this range.

40% and Over

For men, everyday activities are hard to perform and this is where the body fat level approaches morbid obesity. The stomach continues to grow and now the chest is gaining fat.

For women, the thighs and the hips become the outlet of fat and they grow very large. At this level, the waist is usually thirty-five inches or more.

Estimate Calorie Expenditure and Activity Level

Estimating your energy expenditure. This gives the calculator the idea of how much the minimum amount of calories the body will burn every day by calculating the BMR and TEF.

You'll be estimating your activity level. This gives a more realistic look how many calories your body burns.

Then you'll be making the decision on whether you need to lose or gain. For weight gain, a 10-15% calorie is common. For weight loss, any more than a 20% deficit will be very challenging and may be difficult to stick with.

NOTE- You'll also need to keep your carbohydrate intake below thirty grams a day and your protein between 0.7g and 1.2 grams per pound of lean body weight.

Lastly, you'll be given your macros. This is what you need to eat throughout the day. You need to spread this number out.

Example

John is 5'11" and 180 pounds. He lives a lightly active lifestyle. For Keto Diet, John enters all his information into the keto calculator. It recommends he consumes 1695 calories a day with 25g of carbohydrates, 77g of protein, and 143g of fat.

Bottom Line: Use the keto calculator and determine your macros. Based on YOUR macros, you will design your Keto meal plan.

The benefits of a ketogenic diet, are that you'll lose a significant amount of weight, without suffering the hunger pangs sometimes associated with other diets. Your body will burn a decent amount of fat. Your blood sugar will be stabilised because you won't be consuming carbohydrates for energy which makes your blood sugar fluctuate, and instead there's a slow and steady burning of fat. There will be less inflammation in your body, which is good for joint issues, but also skin issues, such as acne. Your hormones will be well regulated, which will mean that your mood will be stable and less prone to swings.

A Ketogenic diet is about eating real food that is good for you. Things like: meat, vegetables, nuts, yoghurts, eggs, and some fruit. It's important to avoid foods that are high in carbohydrates, but also avoid processed foods which contain many preservatives and colourings that just aren't good for you. On a ketogenic diet, it's fine for you to eat beef, lamb, venison and goat, it's best if you can eat animals that have been grass-fed. Red meat such as steak, and ham is good; also, bacon, chicken and turkey. You can eat fatty wild-caught fish and seafood; fish such as salmon, trout, mackerel and tuna. It's best to avoid fish that have been farmed. You can eat pasteurised pork, and poultry and eggs. It's fine to eat gelatine, ghee, butter, and offal which has again come from grass fed animals; organs such as liver, heart and kidneys. It is best to avoid sausages, and avoid meat that has a bread-crumb coating, because the bread crumbs obviously contain carbohydrates.

On a Ketogenic diet, you're able to eat certain fats in abundance, which kind of goes against most people's notion of being on a diet, where usually people hear about 'low fat' products, and desire to get rid of fat off their body. But, on a ketogenic diet saturated fats are permitted, these include: lard, tallow, chicken fat, duck fat, goose fat, clarified butter, ghee, butter, and coconut oil. These also include monounsaturated from items like avocado, macadamia nuts and olive oil. Polyunsaturated omega 3s from things like fatty fish and seafood are very good for you, and are supposed to boost your concentration, clarity and ability to remember and recall. Unprocessed cheese such as cheddar, mozzarella, goat's cheese, cream cheese and blue cheese are all good on this diet.

With regards to vegetables that can be eaten, leafy greens such as spinach, kale, Swiss chard, and radicchio are always good options. Other vegetables include asparagus, squash, celery and bamboo.

If you want a bit of variation in your diet, there are other foods that you can eat occasionally, but not often: cabbage, cauliflower, broccoli, brussels, swede, tomatoes, onions, peppers, leek, mushrooms, pumpkins, squash, berries.

If you require sweeteners in your food and drink, there are sweeteners which are more natural and healthier for you, such as Stevia, or Erythritol. One of the most worrying sweeteners to avoid is aspartame, if you're under any doubt about this, simply do an Internet search about the detrimental side-effects of aspartame, it's in quite a lot of drinks, and candy products, so do be careful to ensure you're not consuming this.

Choose healthy oils, such as extra virgin olive oil, coconut oil, and avocado oil. Avocados generally are very good for you, as well as tasting delicious.

If you need to use cocoa or dark chocolate in your cooking, then the higher the cocoa content the better, aim to pick chocolate that is between 70-90% cocoa and this is much better for you.

Key advice Is that it's best to base your diet mostly on whole, single food ingredients such as meat, fish, eggs, nuts, avocadoes, and low carbohydrate vegetables.

Choose the full fat version of things such as cream, and cheese. This is better for you, than reduced or low-fat products.

Diet Plan

Here's an example below, of what you could eat on a ketogenic diet over the course of a week.

Monday:

Breakfast: Omelette with peppers, onion, avocado and herbs

Lunch: Prawn salad, with avocado and olive oil dressing

Tea: meatballs with cheddar cheese and vegetables

Tuesday:

Breakfast: Strawberry milkshake – see the 5 ingredient recipe in Chapter 10

Lunch: Handful of nuts, celery sticks, avocado and salsa.

Tea: Burger (without a bread-bun) with bacon, egg and cheese.

Wednesday:

Breakfast: Sugar-free yoghurt, with cocoa powder, peanut butter and stevia to sweeten.

Lunch: Milkshake, with almond milk, cocoa powder, peanut butter, and sweetened with stevia.

Tea: Mediterranean pork chops, with parmesan cheese, broccoli and salad – see the 1 ingredient recipe in Chapter 10.

Thursday:

Breakfast: Fried eggs with bacon and mushrooms

Lunch: Ham and cheese slices with nuts.

Tea: Steak and eggs, with a side salad.

Friday:

Breakfast: Ham and cheese pockets (see 5 Ingredient recipe in Chapter 10)

Lunch: Burger with cheese, and salsa.

Tea: Salmon with asparagus cooked in butter

Saturday:

Breakfast: Omelette containing egg, tomato, goat's cheese, and basil.

Lunch: Chicken salad, with olive oil dressing and feta cheese

Tea: White fish, with egg and spinach, cooked in coconut oil.

Sunday:

Breakfast: Bacon, eggs and tomatoes

Lunch: Beef stir fry cooked in coconut oil, with vegetables.

Tea: Chicken stuffed with pesto and cream cheese, with vegetables.

A Side Effect of Ketosis

Losing Weight

Clearly one of the key side effects of ketosis, is the reason that many people embark on a ketogenic, and this is to have rapid weight loss. A low carb diet can be particularly effective for a year to two years, after this time your body become acclimatized to this type of diet, and you may wish to alternate to a different type of diet at this point, for example eating more green food; or trying a diet with lots of juices/smoothies; or moving to a Mediterranean diet is quite a nice option. A Ketogenic diet has been proven to be more effective for people to lose weight, than following a low-fat diet and it's possible to lose 2-3 times as much weight, compared to a low-fat diet.

Lack of Hunger

On many diets people feel hungry; their tummy's rumble and groan and all they can think about all day long is food and when their next meal or snack will be. People the feel irritable and grumpy, and often cease to remain on their diet. When you stop eating so many carbohydrates, you'll immediately become less hungry and will require fewer calories.

The food you eat on a ketogenic diet is good wholesome and filling food.

Loss of Tummy Weight in particular

On a Ketogenic diet, you will find that you'll lose weight from around your abdomen area, which will mean you'll have a flatter tummy. Weight that gathers around the abdominal area is known as 'visceral fat' - this is fat that has attached itself around your vital organs, and this can cause inflammation and 'metabolic dysfunction'. When you go on a Ketogenic, low carbohydrate diet, this has very good results at getting rid of the weight from around your tummy. This will mean that you're at less risk long-term of developing heart disease and Type 2 diabetes.

Improvement to medical conditions

We've seen in the above chapters, that various medical conditions can be greatly improved by following a ketogenic diet. Medical conditions such as epilepsy, high blood pressure, and diabetes. It can help lower cholesterol, and lower high blood pressure, which we'll look at in some later chapters.

Triglycerides Reduce

When triglycerides are present in a high volume in the blood, this is strong indicator that you're at a strong risk of heart disease. The main cause of triglycerides are carbohydrates, and often from fructose. When people cut down their carbohydrate intake, the triglycerides in their blood will reduce dramatically.

HDL Cholesterol Increases

There's much more about this in Chapter 7 of this book, but the key take-away here, is that HDL takes away bad cholesterol from your body and takes it to the liver, where it is re-used or got rid of. If you have HDL, you're at less risk of heart-disease which is clearly a good thing. You can get more HDL by eating fat; and a Ketogenic diet is based upon 75% fat. Eating a ketogenic diet, is therefore much better for you, than eating a low fat diet.

Reduction in Blood Sugar and Insulin Levels

See Chapter 8 for more information about this, but essentially when we eat carbohydrates, this is broken down by our body into digestible sugars, mostly glucose. The more carbohydrates we eat, the more our blood sugar level rises, when we have high blood sugar, this is actually toxic to us, so the pancreas creates insulin which tells the cells to either burn the glucose for fuel for the body, or store it. When we're healthy our pancreas works fine to regulate our sugar. But, many people in the population have a condition known as 'insulin resistance' and cells don't have the insulin input, which can lead to Diabetes. 300 million people have Type 2 Diabetes and this figure is expected to rise. When you cut carbohydrates out of your diet, there's no need for insulin, and you'll find that your blood sugar and insulin levels naturally go down. For people with diabetes who embark on a ketogenic diet, there insulin (with proper medical guidance and advice) 'could' be cut by 50% after just one day on the diet. It is important for diabetics to speak with a Dr, before embarking on a ketogenic diet, but it could certainly be worth doing

Lowers High Blood Pressure

The very fact that your likely to lose weight on a ketogenic diet, is going to help with your high blood pressure. But, research has shown that a Ketogenic diet can be even more effective at lowering blood pressure levels. With experiments that have been carried out, people who have followed a Ketogenic diet have either had their medication drastically reduced for high blood pressure, or they've been able to come off the medication all together.

Combats the Metabolic Syndrome

When people have Metabolic Syndrome, they experience a group of symptoms simultaneously. These include: raised blood pressure, raised blood sugar levels; high triglycerides; low HDL levels; weight gathering around the abdomen. All of these symptoms reduce dramatically once people start to eat a Ketogenic diet. Many people think that a 'low fat' diet is the best, but this doesn't actually address the metabolic issues described here, but ketosis does!

Improvements to LDL Cholesterol

Research has proven that people with high level LDL (Low Density Lipoprotein – sometimes given the name 'bad cholesterol') are much more likely to have a heart attack. The more small cholesterol particles your blood contains the worse this is for risk of heart disease, as these particles stick and fur up arteries; whereas the bigger larger fluffier types of cholesterol are far less harmful, see Chapter 7 for more information about this. Ketogenic diets are able to turn the small troublesome type of cholesterol into bigger less risk particles.

Recovery from Brain Disorders

Ketogenic Diets have been used for a large number of years now, to help children with epilepsy. Especially if epilepsy medication has proven ineffective. A Ketogenic diet has shown that children had 50% less seizures when eating a Ketogenic diet, and 16% of the children had no seizures at all. Ketogenic diets are also effective for those with Dementia and Alzheimer's.

With any kind of medication, drug, herb, diet, exercise regime you will get good side effects, and some people may experience 'some' less positive side-effects. These have been included in the book here, not to put you off the Ketogenic diet, as we firmly believe that the Ketogenic diet is excellent, and will improve your overall health. But, we've included the list below, as some people (especially in the first couple of weeks when the diet is new), 'may' experience some of the following. They've been included here, so that if you experience them, you know it's ok, and it's not uncommon, and also some ideas of what to do to combat them. 2 of the key things to keep in mind, are that any less positive side-effects you experience will be drastically improved if you increase your water consumption and keep flushing things through your body; also adding a little more pink Himalayan rock salt to your diet may help, and finally, give the diet a bit of time and let your body adjust to it, and with time, you'll find that any less positive side-effects will dissipate and you'll be left with just good results!

Less positive side-effects

Some of the less favourable side-effects of Ketosis, are symptoms which you may experience with pretty much any diet, whereby you're reducing your intake of a substance you used to consume. So, if you're eating less sugar, and less carbohydrates, your body is detoxing from these chemicals that you'd usually consume. Some of the side-effects you 'could' experience, are headaches; fatigue; constipation or diarrhoea; general lethargy and weakness; and bad breath. Depending on how strict your diet is, you may need to ensure that you're getting enough of all the vital vitamins and minerals you require.

When ketosis occurs, what is actually happening is that your body has run out of sugar (glucose) which gives you energy. So, instead it starts to break down fat, in order to give you the energy your require. When this takes place, ketones are built up inside you.

Researchers have postulated that if people continue to eat a low carb diet, and eat lots of protein and fat, this may pose a risk of heart disease developing, and the risk of certain cancers also increases too.

Leg Cramps

Another side-effect that could occur on a low-carb diet, is leg-cramps. This may be, because of the change in diet, you urinate more, and therefore lose some minerals such as magnesium. Again the answer is to drink salty drinks, such as broth and bouillon. You could also consider take a magnesium food supplement (tablet) from a health food shop, on its own or part of a daily multivitamin and mineral tablet.

A key solution to many of the side-effects experienced in the first week or two of a low carb diet, is to increase how much water you drink, and also to up the salt you consume (unless you have high blood pressure, where increasing your salt would be dangerous to your health). A nice way to do both at once, can sometimes to have a savoury drink, such as Bovril, which will give you both liquid and salt. You can start to do this, a week before you start a low carb diet, and that may prevent any of the negative side-effects.

Bad Breath

When you enter ketosis, this may change the way that your breath smells. Your breath may smell a mixture between fruity, and like acetone nail-polish remover. This is because acetone is a ketone. This shows that your body has changed from burning carbohydrates for energy, to burning fat as your body's fuel instead. The same smell may come from pores in your skin, and when you sweat when you exercise or exert yourself. This won't happen with everyone on a ketogenic diet, and if it does occur, it will usually only last for a couple of weeks. You need to ensure that your mouth has plenty of moisture in it, by drinking enough water. Brush your teeth at least twice a day, this won't really impact on the fruity acetone smell, as this comes from your lungs, but by maintaining good oral hygiene the fruity smell won't be mixed with whatever you've eaten. You can regularly use a breath freshner and mouth wash, to disguise the fruity smell. It's sensible to pursue your ketogenic diet and put up with this for a couple of weeks, as usually after that time, it will have naturally passed. As a last resort, you could decide to come out of the state of ketosis. Eating 50-70g of carbohydrates a day, would do this. However, if you come out of ketosis, then your body will not continue to burn fat instead of carbohydrates. You could decide to do a diet that has some fasting in it, and this may reduce the fruity breath occurring.

Constipation

If you experience constipation on a low carb diet, there are several things you can do to help this. It's not unusual to experience constipation at first, simply because you've changed your diet, and are no longer eating as many carbohydrates, and your body will need to adjust to this, and your digestive system get back into the flow of things. Usually, when we're constipated, this is because we don't have enough fluid in our gut, to keep things moving smoothly and food becomes, dry, hard and gets stuck and will create discomfort in your stomach. So, an easy answer is simply to drink a lot more water. When you drink more, your intestines find it easier to absorb water from your food to aid digestion. Ensure you eat plenty of vegetables, and citrus fruits. You can also eat fruits, such as prunes which have a mild laxative effect. Eat food which is a source of fibre, or take food supplements such as psyllium husks which you can dissolve in water. Finally, if none of the above works (and the key one really is drinking a lot more water), then you could take some over the counter medicine from your pharmacy, such as milk of magnesia.

Heavy cold symptoms

When you start a ketogenic diet, you can expect to feel a little like you've come down with a heavy cold; this is sometimes known as 'induction flu' because the symptoms feel similar, with headaches, feeling sick, feeling tired and lethargic. You can feel like your head is muzzy, and unable to think as quickly and clearly as is usual for you. Don't worry, this won't last. You may feel a bit bad tempered and irritable. This is because you may feel deprived from your carbs, and whenever we feel like we're missing out on something that we'd like to eat, it's natural that we initially feel a bit grumpy about this. People have spoken about diets making them feel like Jekyll and Hyde, where they know that they need to cut out or cut down on certain foods in order to become healthier; yet at the very same time, they're mardy about doing so, and feel annoyed by the fact that they can't eat exactly what they want; there's the eternal battle of a devil on one shoulder, and an angel on the other; good vs. evil.

If you want to succeed with any diet you need to push through this stage, and just accept that your body is getting rid of any toxins, adapting to a new way of working without so many carbohydrates, and that this stage will not last forever, and that if you stick with it, you will feel considerably better and see good results.

I can't emphasize enough that drinking plenty of water is the key to eliminating symptoms like this quickly. You can also drink things like chicken stock, bouillon, or bone broth to give you a bit of salt, and a better taste to what you're drinking.

When you're on a low carb diet, it is important that you eat fat. You are allowed to eat things like butter. Your body will just be adapting to change throughout this phase, as it's changing from what it's been used to most of its life, ie. Burning carbohydrates for energy; changing to burning fat for energy instead. It's a big difference, but worth the results.

A final option when you're trying to achieve ketosis, but dislike any side effects, is to introduce just a very small amount of carbs. But, this should be done as a last resort really. Because it will take you longer to achieve ketosis if you're still eating carbohydrates. Doing this, would also slow down any health benefits.

Tips for Success with Keto Diet

There are a few things that you need to know before you embark on the ketogenic diet. Below are 9 tips to help you be successful with this diet.

Tip #1: Count Carbohydrates

There are some useful apps out there you can find on your phone or online calculators to count net carbohydrates. However, there is a simple way to do this. When in doubt, simply take the total carbohydrates listed on a product's label and subtract the fiber from that total amount. This is your net carbohydrates. Of course, if you're eating fresh, whole foods, this is a little more difficult because there isn't any label packaging. That's where apps are handy.

Tip #2: Planning and Preparation

Planning for this diet, you need to shop for the right foods and cook at home more. Creating and following a meal plan is key to success. Sit down and outline your day/week/month, and don't forget to plan for snacks!

Tip #3: Eat Enough Fat

With this diet, fat makes up 70% of your caloric intake. That's a lot of fat. In order to get enough calories, stock up on the fat. Even if you are in a calorie deficit, you're still eating 70% fat. If you're having trouble getting enough fat, stock up on the olive oil, coconut oil and butter. You'll be eating a lot of these fats, bulk purchase to save money.

Tip #4: Make Keto a Lifestyle

It's a good idea to try turning the ketogenic diet into a lifestyle plan. This means making the diet into a habit. In order to do this, you need to first try not to overwhelm yourself and don't get upset if you backpedal and don't follow the plan. Immediately return to it and try again.

Commitment is key! Commit to the ketogenic diet for a week, two weeks, and then maybe a month. By the end of a month, it will turn into a habit and living this new lifestyle won't seem as difficult.

Tip #5: Drink Plenty of Water

Entering a stage of ketosis will naturally deplete your body's water supply. Therefore, you need to drink tons of water in order to stay hydrated, but not only that, you need to keep an eye on your electrolyte levels, too.

Tip #6: Increase Salt Intake

As levels of insulin circulating through your body lower, your kidneys will begin excreting some excess sodium. Eat more salt to avoid electrolyte deficiency.

Tip #7: Experiment

Have fun with this diet! Although there are restrictions, compared to most diets, it's flexible and so delicious. Play around with recipes and different ingredients. Enjoy trying new foods you might have never explored, just make sure you're following your macros.

Tip #8: Keto + Intermittent Fasting

A common practice for rapid weight loss is combining ketogenic diet with intermittent fasting. This is common as many people find it easier and more convenient to meet their macros with this pattern of eating. Intermittent fasting involves cycles between periods of fasting (fasted state) and eating (fed state)

Tip #9: Patience

Be patient. Follow the diet, and the results will show over time. Don't stress out if results don't show up immediately. Good things come to those who are disciplined and have patience. Eating more carbs will be tempting, if you really want the results, stick to your macros.

What to Avoid on the Ketogenic Diet?

Because Ketosis can be actively measured as to the state that your metabolism is at, it is perfectly possible to state whether foods can or can't be eaten on this diet.

It's possible for you to eat foods that you think will put you into a state of Ketosis (this is covered in the next chapter) and then test your ketone levels.

You need to be avoiding carbohydrates, so it's best to avoid all grains, and in with this, that obviously covers things such as bread, pizza dough, pasta, crackers, and cookies. Avoid sugar, sweets, cakes, syrups and soft drinks that have a vast amount of sugar in them. Avoid soda, fruit juice, smoothies that you have bought and not made yourself (green smoothies you've made are acceptable); avoid fruit (small portions of berries are ok; and ½ a Granny Smith apple in a green smoothie). Avoid beans and legumes, things like peas, chickpeas, lentils and kidney beans. Avoid root vegetables, such as potatoes, carrots, parsnips. Try to avoid sauces, things like ketchup and brown sauce and many salad dressings often contain a lot of sugar and unhealthy fats. Try to limit the amount of mayonnaise you have, and vegetable oil.

Avoid products that are labelled as 'low fat' - most of these will contain sugars and starches. When you're buying meat, look for meat and poultry that is grass or grain fed, rather than farmed, as farmed meat and poultry is high in omega 6s. If you buy farmed fish, that may contain PCBs or mercury, all of which is dangerous and damaging to health. If you buy bacon, you need to be aware of preservatives and added starches. If you want brazil nuts, try not to eat too many of them because they contain very high levels of selenium.

Processed foods are to be avoided, because they may contain MSG, sulphites and carrageenan, they may also contain wheat and gluten.

There are a number of fruits that it's best to avoid, or to really eat tiny amounts of when you're on a ketogenic diet. These include: peaches and nectarines, apples, oranges, plums, kiwis, fresh figs, apricots, grapefruits, cherries, pears and dragon fruits.

If you're trying hard to lose weight, then you really should avoid alcohol entirely. However, if you've reached a stage where you're happy with the weight you are, and you're just wanting to remain at that weight, then you are able to drink red or white wine, that is dry, rather than sweet.
Refined fats and oils are to be avoided, as well as trans fats such as margarine. Refined fats and oils include: sunflower, soybean, canola, corn oil and grapeseed.

Milk is not recommended to be consumed, because most of the 'goodness' in the milk has been removed via the process of pasteurisation. It's quite high in carbohydrates. It's recommended that you replace milk with cream in drinks where you're able to. For alternative to dairy milk, you could try nut milks instead, such as almond or coconut. Instead of grain flours you can use nut flours too, such as almond or coconut flour.

Avoid sugar-free diet food. These can often contain sugar-alcohol which can impact upon your ketone levels. These types of food are often highly processed, and some of them too can cause a laxative effect.

Fruit juices are best to be avoided, even fruit juices that claim to be 100% fruit juice; because fruit juices are naturally very sugary, smoothies are slightly more acceptable because they contain more fibre, but you would be better off just drinking pure water.

Avoid potatoes; avoid processed food such as burgers; avoid beans and soy products; avoid dried fruit and processed biscuits and sweets; avoid grains and gluten.

How to Reach a State of Ketosis?

Ketosis is where your metabolism can be physically measured. So, it's not just a general idea or method, it is something which can be scientifically proven as to whether you are in a state of ketosis or not. You can opt to eat foods that you think will put you into a state of ketosis, and then test your ketone levels.

When people eat a high fat and low carbohydrate diet, as in a Ketogenic diet, the body runs out of sugary glucose to use as fuel for energy. So, your liver starts to break down fatty acids, which provide fuel to the body muscles, heart tissue and brain and this is what is known as ketosis. This is the key reason that people embark on a ketogenic diet, in order to reach this state.

The ketones in your body contain the following and these are water-soluble and released when ketosis occurs:

- acetone (whilst you may have seen the ingredient acetone in nail-varnish remover and paint thinners, it is also a product that occurs naturally within the body). Acetone is created when acetoacetate breaks down. Acetone enters the lungs and is expelled when you breath out. This is why people sometimes say that when people are in a state of ketosis their breath has a fruity chemical smell, it is acetone that causes this. It is this acetone on the breath that can be measured to determine how far into ketosis a person is; the more acetone, the further the level of ketosis. You can measure acetone in other ways, you can check levels of it in urine and in blood too. You can test your urine with a urine strip that will change colour to alert you to your level of ketosis, this is an OK method, but not 100% accurate. It is an affordable technique. You can have a blood test, that will measure the glucose in your blood, this is highly accurate, but is very expensive and most people aren't terribly keen on having their blood tested. You can get a Ketonix breath measurer, and this is fairly affordable, it's again not 100% accurate, but not a bad way to measure acetone from your lungs. If you use a breath monitor and the result is between 40-80 that would usually indicate that you're in a state of Ketosis. Once you have bought a breath metre, it's a one-off payment and you're then able to continue to use that breath metre for the rest of your life, unlike urine strips which you'd need to replace when you run out; or the fairly complex invasive procedure of having blood taken by a medical person.

- **acetoacetate** – this is the product that will be created first, when you enter a state of Ketosis.

- betahydroxybutryate – this is the product that is created second after acetoacetate when you've entered the state of ketosis.

It's important not to confuse Ketosis (which is a desirable state to reach) with Ketoacidosis (DKA) which is something that can occur in people with the condition Type 1 Diabetes, or it can occur sometimes in people who are alcoholics. Ketosis is a safe state for people to be in who are following a ketogenic diet. Please don't be scared off a Ketogenic diet, by people who are misinformed and are confusing it, with the diabetic condition of ketoacidosis – the names are slightly similar so it's easy to see the confusion, but these are very different things. When you're in Ketosis, this is a normal healthy metabolic state and you'll have between 1-5 mmol ketones in your blood. Ketoacidosis which is something else entirely, a dangerous metabolic state, affects people with diabetes, is where you'd have excessive levels of ketones in your blood, usually 15-30 mmol ketones. Ketoacidosis can often occur in Type 1 diabetics, simply due to how much processed food, containing carbohydrates, people eat. If you don't have Diabetes, it's physically impossible for your body to go into ketoacidosis. Ketosis and Ketoacidosis are two separate words, and two very different things, that should not be confused.

In order to reach a state of Ketosis, you need to remember to keep eating fats, and really limit your carbohydrate intake. Having 75% fat; 20% protein and only 5% carbohydrate are the key figures to keep in mind when you're planning your daily food intake. If you keep eating like this, drinking water and exercising, with time, your WILL achieve ketosis.

Improved cholesterol readings

Some people may mistakenly believe that because you're eating a high fat diet, you'll have high cholesterol. This is not the case. Research has proven that low carbohydrate diets, actually can give you good cholesterol levels and give you a healthy heart. Our bodies contain fatty acids which are actually good for us. One of these fatty acids are known as triglycerides. Triglycerides can be used as energy, and broken down into glucose. If you have too much glucose in your blood this could lead you to develop diabetes or heart disease, or other diseases.

Our bodies naturally produce 75% of the cholesterol we have; and the remaining 25% of our cholesterol is from the food we eat. HDL Cholesterol in our bodies, is not actually cholesterol, but it's something that transports cholesterol in our body. It's commonly called 'good cholesterol' but it is just a means of transportation of cholesterol to the liver where it is destroyed. When it is destroyed, this then stops the cholesterol furring up arteries and prevents blockages. HDL cholesterol therefore is healthy, and people with low levels of HDL cholesterol are at greater risk of heart disease. Research has shown that people with a carbohydrate restricted diet (like on a ketogenic diet) have double to amount of HDL cholesterol compared to those on other diets. If people eat less than 20g of Carbohydrates per day, then that can increase the HDL cholesterol by four times as much!

LDL is the bad type of cholesterol that can contribute towards heart disease.

A 2004 research study by Dashti and Matthew et al, into *The Longterm Effects of a Ketogenic Diet in Obese Patients* found that people lost weight, and that their body-mass index decreased, and that their cholesterol decreased also over the 24 weeks of the study.

Many people think that the best thing to lower cholesterol levels would be to eat a low-fat diet, and this couldn't be more wrong! The best thing to lower your cholesterol is to reduce your carbohydrate intake. Foods like butter, meat and cheese are good for you, and should be part of your diet. Our bodies need cholesterol and naturally make cholesterol in your brain, liver, and most of your body's cells. Cholesterol is crucial to how bile, vitamin D and sex hormones are created in your body. Cholesterol allows substances to be transported through your body. If you have high cholesterol this doesn't necessarily mean you're a prime candidate for heart disease. Many people with 'normal' levels of cholesterol still have heart attacks, whilst many people with high cholesterol are perfectly healthy.

Some have argued that the 'good' and 'bad' cholesterol types are considered dated now, but instead that it's necessary to look at the type and size of the cholesterol. It's important to know how many type A and type B particles you have. When you have sticky dense cholesterol that sticks to lining of your blood vessels this is often caused by too much glucose in your blood, which again points to too many carbohydrates. Type A particles are the best type to have in your cholesterol, and you can get more of these by eating good fats. Type B particles are the bad type of cholesterol from sugar. You need to eat more fat, and less sugar, which is why a Ketogenic diet is perfect. When you eat a lot of sugar, your artery walls narrow, and work with the kidneys to retain water, in order to tray and dilute how much sugar there is in your blood. The more sugar you eat, the more triglycerides you'll have in your blood and this does put you at greater risk of heart disease.

What you need to avoid in your body is inflammation. This is the leading cause of heart disease. Cholesterol can cause inflammation, but only when cholesterol is damaged and of the B Type that sticks. Eating a high carbohydrate diet, having high insulin levels, eating processed food which contains salt, sugars, preservatives, being under stress, and drinking too much alcohol, and smoking all contribute towards inflammation in your body.

If your cholesterol levels are very low, this isn't actually a good thing. We're taught so much that cholesterol is bad, but this isn't the case! If your cholesterol levels are low, then you're susceptible to things like Alzheimer's disease, depression, feeling suicidal, and acting in an aggressive manner. Statins that lower cholesterol can impact upon your memory, as well as causing leg-pains. You're encouraged to eat Omega 3 fats because these reduce inflammation, whereas Omega 6 fats cause inflammation. Omega 3 fats include wild fish, macadamia nuts, walnuts, grass-fed meat, and flax seeds. Omega 6 fats include vegetable oil, canola oil and soy oil – these should be avoided. Wherever possible avoid statins and these can cause more damage than good to your health; they can also cause diabetes and lower your immune system. Statins also affect your ability to produce hormones, bile and vitamin D. If you eat a low fat, and wholegrain diet thinking that you're being healthy, you're actually not helping your heart at all. The best thing you can do is stick to good, real nutritious food, which is low carbohydrate, high fat, and unprocessed. The belief that fat makes you fat, is actually unfounded.

Reduction in blood sugar and blood pressure

Insulin is what regulates your blood sugar in your body. This is why people with diabetes, sometimes have insulin injections. A ketogenic diet can reduce your blood sugar, and help to bring down triglycerides and glucose in your blood to a more manageable level. Insulin is created in the pancreas; the pancreas also assists the digestive system by creating enzymes. Insulin works to metabolize carbohydrates and fats, and carbohydrates as we know well by know contain a lot of sugars, and these are broken down into glucose. This gives you a certain amount of energy; which is why you often find glucose in energy drinks, or glucose energy tablets. Insulin works to help cells in the body absorb the glucose and this in itself helps to reduce the amount of glucose in the bloodstream. When we eat, due to what we consume (especially when it's carbohydrates) our blood sugar goes up; at this point the pancreas releases insulin which should help your liver, muscles and fat to absorb with glucose from your blood. In people without Diabetes, the body should work to keep these blood sugar levels normal.

With modern diets today, many people have an imbalance of glucose and insulin in their bodies and in particular insulin-resistance occurs and your cells don't react in the way they should to insulin. If your cells keep building up this resistance to insulin, your pancreas won't be able to cope with this. If the glucose can't be absorbed from your bloodstream, your pancreas will be unable to make the insulin required and you'll have too much glucose in your blood, which can result in diabetes and metabolic syndrome, which are a few conditions grouped together that can include: increased blood pressure, high blood sugar, an increase in body fat, especially around the waist, and out of range cholesterol or triglyceride levels; all of these conditions appear to occur simultaneously and can increase your chances of getting heart disease, strokes and diabetes. Almost a quarter of the population are thought to have insulin resistance, but many people are unaware of this, until they develop Diabetes. If you are overweight, smoke, have known heart-disease, don't exercise, have high blood pressure, have high cholesterol, or polycystic ovary syndrome, or belong to certain ethnic groups which are more prone to diabetes, then it can be worth getting tested every 2-3yrs if you're over the age of 45.

Whilst there is medication that can assist in regulating diabetes, one of the best treatments for diabetes is to change your lifestyle. If you can lose weight, and exercise more, then your body will become more able to use insulin correctly once again. Smoking causes problems with insulin, so if you're a smoker, it really would be in your best interest to try to stop (or severely cut down). It clearly would make good sense to reduce your carbohydrate intake too and this is the whole purpose of the ketogenic diet. In a 2005 experiment to test how effective the ketogenic diet is at improving insulin levels, the research found that after just 2 weeks of following a ketogenic diet, the subject's insulin levels improved by 75%. Other research studies have looked at comparing low fat diets, with a high fat ketogenic diet. Whilst the diets, led to similar weight loss, the ketogenic diet did yield much better results with regards to insulin. So, if your insulin levels are high, or you're insulin resistant, a low carbohydrate diet can be really effective.

If you have high blood pressure (also known as hypertension) this can increase the likelihood of you contracting many diseases, including heart disease, stroke, and kidney failure. Eating a ketogenic diet reduces your blood pressure, and this will reduce the risk of you contracting these diseases and will give you more longevity.

Other Benefits of a Ketogenic Diet

Following a ketogenic diet, can help you in so many different ways. It can help you lose weight, help revert diabetes, give you much greater mental focus, make you more able to participate in physical activity, it can help with the symptoms of epilepsy and make this more controllable and suppress seizures, it can make your blood pressure stabilize, it can reduce the symptoms of acne, it can reduce heart-burn, it can aid your digestive system and give you less symptoms of bloating, gurgling, upset tummies. The diet can help with heart disease. The diet can help those who have experience brain injuries, such as concussion. The diet will reduce sugar cravings, which again will aid you to lose weight if you're not wanting to eat as much sweet food.

With regards to Diabetes (which is caused by high blood sugar and insulin not working correctly in the body) – a ketogenic diet can help you to lose weight. With people who have Type 2 diabetes, being overweight is often a key factor. Eating a ketogenic diet can improve insulin sensitivity by 75%, which is just tremendous. 1/3 of diabetic people who start a ketogenic diet, can come off medication all together, and 95% of others are able to really reduce the amount of medication that they take.

If you have Polycystic Ovary Syndrome (PCOS) this can cause menstrual problems, plus other issues such as acne, weight gain, an increase in body hair, and even including infertility. Eating a low-carb diet can really help to reverse the symptoms of PCOS. PCOS is common in women who have Type II diabetes, and we've already discussed how a Ketogenic diet can assist with Type II diabetes earlier in the book. There is a lot of evidence to suggest that PCOS can be caused by high insulin levels. If women with PCOS lose weight, this has been proven to have beneficial effects. A low carb diet will lower insulin levels, and will help you to lose weight. In studies that have been conducted, women with PCOS who followed a low carb diet did lose weight, had reduced body hair, felt better hormonally, and half of the group who had previously had infertility problems did become pregnant too. In comparison to just using medication, having a ketogenic diet has increased the chances of a person becoming pregnant from 45% to over 90%. This means that many people don't require IV treatment.

It's been suggested that a Ketogenic Diet 'could' assist those with Epilepsy. Now, if you or a family members/friend has epilepsy, we would of course only suggest that you follow a ketogenic diet under strict medical guidance, and we would never suggest that this diet should be a replacement for medication that the person with epilepsy is on. But, it is certainly worth researching further and speaking with your medical advisers to seek their opinion on the matter.

The ketogenic diet has also been shown to help with other conditions such as Alzheimer's, Parkinsons, and even some types of cancer. Whereas healthy cells can use the ketones and create energy out of them; cancer cells aren't able to do this and cancer cells die off because they don't have anything to help them live and regenerate. A trial took place in 2011 with patients who had advanced cancer. Cancerous tumours use glucose for energy and fuel. So, giving cancer patients a diet that has good fat and protein, but limits carbohydrates that the tumours thrive on and use to grow, is a good technique. The patients' ketone levels were measured in their urine. Some of the patients did not feel able to stick to the diet, but out of the patients who did, reported no negative side-effects of the diet, and that they felt emotionally better and suffered less from insomnia. In children with cancer, a ketogenic diet has had excellent results. A ketogenic diet, also seems effective in inhibiting tumour cell growth in colon and breast cancer. A ketogenic diet had been shown to decrease tumour growth and increase survival time.

Keto-lifestyle and a complete two-week meal plan.

Basics of a Ketogenic diet plan

Low carbohydrate diets are quite common, but they certainly don't follow the principles of a ketogenic diet plan. Most individuals may confuse a ketogenic diet plan with a regular low carbohydrate, high protein ketogenic diet. The ketogenic diet plan has completely different allowances of carbohydrate, fat and protein, and we have broken down the basics for you:

- The basic and most important principle of a ketogenic diet plan is to limit the amount of carbohydrate intake daily, and reduce it to not more than 20-60 grams per day. The trick is to keep a count the amount of carbohydrate you are consuming on a daily basis. This is necessary to attain a state of ketosis in your body, where the glucose levels will reduce and fats, that is, ketone bodies will become the primary source of fuel. For beginners, less than 100 grams of carbs per day is a good option, but is still a high amount for a ketogenic diet. Hence, the amount of carbs has to be reduced gradually.

- A low carb diet does not mean that the loss can be overcome by high protein amounts, as too much amount is bound to hamper the mechanism of ketosis, and hence, the true essence of a ketogenic diet. The ideal protein intake should be determined by calculated one's ideal body weight, based on his/her height. The remaining calories after carbohydrate and protein amounts have been determined should come from fat. This is eventually help in attaining the state of ketosis, which will help one to fully reap the numerous benefits of a ketogenic diet.

- Hence, to sum up the daily calorie intake of an individual consuming a ketogenic diet, 5-10% calories should come from carbohydrates, 20-25% calories should come from proteins and lastly, 70-75% calories should come from fats. The idea is to replace high carbohydrate foods with high fat and moderate protein recipes.

- Why this unusual combination of protein and fat you may ask? Simply because, high levels of fat do not create sudden spikes in sugar and insulin levels, and maintains a steady supply of energy. Protein levels should be essentially moderate, as high levels of protein in a low carb diet, may induce gluconeogenesis, a state in which non-carb sources like proteins are utilized to release glucose. This may spike insulin and glucose levels which may interfere in achieving ketosis in a ketogenic diet.

A complete two-week meal Plan

There are many of you whose New Year Resolution probably may have been about losing weight and to become slim and trim as fast as possible but without the side effects. If this is what you have in mind, then this diet plan is sure to bring plenty of inspiration and motivate you to feel great throughout the year and to consume healthily.

Doing some research will help you to come across a complete list of the available free diet plans that you can follow depending on your specific needs, requirements, moods and taste. There are readily available several diet plans that can be followed by anyone like paleo/keto, primal/keto, vegetarian/keto diet plans, along with meal plan to reduce fat quickly! However, all diet plans do include easy to prepare recipes and shopping list. This way, you can ensure not having to waste your precious time in the kitchen and can get your diet plan ready within minutes.

But, before getting into the new diet plan, there are few frequently asked questions that you need to know about keto diet. This way, you can be better prepared to implement them without any hassle or worry.

Here it is, the satisfying and delicious meal plan to jump start the first fourteen days of your new ketogenic lifestyle. When following this plan, remember that when you eat ketogenically you do not need to overthink portion size or calories. Each recipe has been created to limit carbs while promoting fats and protein. The idea behind the 70:20:10 ratio is to give you a general guideline to help you choose what foods to consume. If your ratios end up a little high or a little low, that is fine. Just remember to keep the total grams of net carbohydrates in a range that puts you in and maintains ketosis throughout these fourteen days. This meal plan has been created to help you eat ketogenically, but also realistically.

Snacks are included at the end of the meal plan. It is important that you consume two to three snacks per day. This will help keep your blood sugar level steady, keep your body fueled, and keep you satisfied. Traditionally, during the first two weeks of a ketogenic diet plan, desserts are not consumed. I know that even though you will be satisfied with the eating plan, emotionally you might still seek something a little sweet. Diets turn into lifestyles only when they work realistically with how we live our lives. For this reason, if you find yourself with a bit of a sweet tooth, try one of the breakfast shakes, a selection of fresh berries and cheese or a square of decadent extra dark chocolate.

Now all you need to do is begin and enjoy!

a) If you're only cooking for yourself, refrigerate or freeze the remaining servings. You could also half your recipes.

b) Feel free to swap your breakfast recipes for lunch, or lunch for dinner in the same day. It's also okay to swap one day's recipe for another.

c) You don't have to take any snacks between meals, but if you absolutely have to, ensure that you take something keto friendly.

d) Very low-carb foods are usually low in magnesium too. I recommend taking some magnesium supplements or snacks that are high in magnesium, like nuts. Also, be sure to take extra sodium; pink Himalayan salt will do

e) The keto buns are to be made much in advance (full 10 recipes can be prepared). Freeze for keeping fresh as well as defrost the night before at room temperature or in the oven before serving.

f) Though I have seen this 14-day keto diet plan help many people kick start their weight loss and healthy living journey in an incredible way, it may not work for everyone. You might need to make small adjustments. In case you need to take less protein, reduce your portions of meat and eggs. However, ensure that you don't neglect proteins completely, as this will prevent you from achieving ketosis.

g) Don't worry about a little extra protein; it won't prevent you from reaching ketosis. On the contrary, it will keep your hunger at bay. In case you need to add or reduce your fat intake, concentrate on the fatty foods and oils when making adjustments.

h) Don't eat when you don't feel hungry, even if you have to skip a meal.

Recipe substitutions

If you are intolerant to certain foods or just hate particular ingredients, here are some options that you can try:

- You can substitute fish, pork, and lamb with one another, as they have a similar nutritional profile

- If you don't take bacon, take beef chorizo or roast beef instead

- You can substitute ultimate keto buns for nut free keto buns

- You can substitute vanilla keto smoothie, chocolate keto smoothie, and pumpkin smoothie with one another

Meal prepping

Meal prepping is sometimes misunderstood. Most people assume you just have to start cooking for a week and that's it. But, it doesn't really work like that. It requires thorough planning, knowing what ingredients to use, what to buy etc. Meal prepping while on a Ketogenic Diet requires a sort of scientific approach. Luckily, no degree is required! Some of the tips include:

1. Create a winning framework by evaluating your eating habits

First, and the most important thing you should consider prior to starting meal prepping, is evaluating you and your family's eating habits. Ideally, you should strive to introduce healthy eating habits to your lifestyle and prepping meals is a marvelous way to start. You're probably wondering why you have to evaluate your eating habits in the first place. The reason is simple – it will give you a direct insight into how much food you should prep, what ingredients to limit or add, etc. Furthermore, evaluating eating habits also shows how healthy or unhealthy your lifestyle is and serves as additional motivation to start with this idea. Here are a few tips you should bear in mind:

- How many meals do you eat per day (together with snacks)? If you're married with kids, how many meals you eat together? Ideally, you should take a notebook and write down answers to these questions for each member of the family. This will give you a rough idea as to how much food you should prepare. It's also useful for measuring portions and portion control.

- How much time do you have to prepare meals for yourself or family members? Does it take too long? Do you have to work late the upcoming week? Will your work hours interfere with cooking time for your family? If you're on the go or have a busy schedule, you should opt for meals that are easy to prepare and safe to spend a few days in the cooler. That way, your family will have the dinner ready and you won't have to spend too much time in the kitchen cooking when all you want to do is to relax.

- Do you find yourself craving certain foods? Does your mood affect decisions about meals you want to cook? Weather changes, seasons, moods, cravings, etc., have a significant impact on your eating habits and therefore on meal prepping as well. This is also something you should consider when planning to prep your meals. For instance, if it's winter, try preparing warm, nutritious, and tasty meals that you and your family will love to eat. Also, if you find yourself craving snacks in between meals, you can also opt for and prepare healthier alternatives.

- Budget – Let's face it: it plays a pivotal role. To impeccably execute meal prepping, you should make sure that your meal plan fits into your budget. To do so, you should determine the amount of money you set out for food, outline your potential meal plan, and see how they fit together. Make sure you don't plan meals that are way over-budget because that won't only affect your financial situation, but will also affect your meal prepping endeavors at the same time.

- As you can see, evaluating eating habits is an extremely practical way of determining how much food you're going to prepare. Here's what else you should do:

- Before you start with prepping meals, keep a journal of all the meals you prepare and eat. After a few days, read everything you wrote and look for patterns that repeat. Are these habits healthy or unhealthy? If unhealthy, that indicates something you should limit or avoid

- Consider how quickly you and your family eat, how much you eat, and how much food you throw away

- Plan your meals with the help of notebook and pen, or put the plan into your smartphone.

2. Shop Smart

Healthy nutrition starts with making wise choices when shopping for groceries. Preparing healthy meals can turn into quite a hassle if you don't have the right ingredients. Meal prepping on a Ketogenic diet won't work if you don't buy the right types of food. When food shopping, always remember the following tips:

Produce – Ideally, you should go for local produce. Since you already know what's in season in your area, it will be easier for you to plan your meals. But, this isn't the only thing you should consider when buying produce. Here's what else you should know:

- Don't always assume that organic produce is more expensive

- Buy in season
- Try to grow your own

Fish – There are multiple reasons to eat fish and if you don't have a habit of including it into your diet, you should definitely do so. Eating fish lowers the risk for strokes and heart attacks. It increases grey matter. Fish may prevent and relieve depression. It's the only good dietary source of much-needed Vitamin D. Regular consumption of fish lowers the risk for autoimmune diseases, Type 2 diabetes, protects eye health, and improves sleep.

When buying fresh steaks or fillets you should look for:

- When purchasing white-fleshed fish you should opt for translucent-looking fillets with pinkish meat
- When buying colored fish (any color) check whether flesh appears dense without any gaps between layers
- In case fish is wrapped in plastic, the package shouldn't contain liquid

When buying frozen fish, remember this:

- Opt for well-sealed packages from the bottom of the freezer case that are old up to 3 months

• Look for shiny, rock-hard frozen fish without freezer-burn spots, ice crystals, or frost.

Red Meat – Just like fish, in order to get the best out of meat you buy, you have to know how to shop for it. Here are a few tips:

• Meat should be well-butchered and cuts shouldn't have ragged edges, uneven sections, or hacked bits

• Colour varies depending on cut or animal, but ideally it should be vibrant and rich instead of dull

• Texture should NOT be loose, uneven, and there shouldn't be broken fibers.

Chicken – Who doesn't like chicken? Some of our favorite meals include yummy chicken, but you can't buy just any piece of chicken there is. Here are some chicken shopping tips that you should employ:

• Fresh chicken is pink

• Stay away from chicken (or poultry in general) with grayish or transparent meat

• Look under crevices, e.g. under wings and thighs, and check for tears in the skin (torn skin also affects quality of meat)

• Avoid bloody chicken

• Press against the chicken; fresh chicken has skin that springs back once you press against it

• Smell it; fresh chicken doesn't have smell.

Eggs – They are incredibly nutritious and it's impossible to have breakfast without them. Here are a few tips for eggs shopping:

• Colour doesn't matter; they are all equally nutritious

• Check the carton for sell-by date. If we assume they are stored properly, eggs are good for consumption between 4 and 6 weeks after this date

• Ensure that the eggs are intact without cracks.

• If you're making meals based on recipes, then go for eggs graded as large because that's the standardized size used when recipes are tested.

3. How to use herbs and spices properly

Herbs and spices have been used for centuries not only for culinary purposes, but for medical purposes as well. They have the ability to offer a wide array of health benefits while enhancing the flavor of the food you eat. In order to enjoy eating delicious meals enriched with herbs and spices, you have to know how to store them properly. That's what we're going to discuss now.

Buying and storing spices:

- Buy whole spices whenever possible – Ground spices lose their potency quite quickly, while whole spices such as cardamom, black pepper, cloves, cinnamon, etc. can be kept up to 2 years and still provide plenty of flavor to your food. Plus, whole spices are more versatile as you can use them as whole, or grind them

- Replenish spices from the bulk section – You already know that spices sold in glass jars are more expensive than spices sold in bulk. When you empty out spices in a glass jar, you can safely opt to replenish the stash with spices from the bulk section. Buying in bulk has numerous benefits including purchasing smaller amounts so you won't throw away spices you don't use frequently and it's needless to mention this option is more beneficial for your budget

- Store spices in a dark and cool place

- Toast and ground spices yourself – why toast? Because it enhances the flavor of spices!

Depending on your needs, you can also buy fresh or dried herbs. Ideally, you should store them in airtight containers and move them away from direct sunlight unless you're buying fresh herbs that you want to dry yourself.

Using herbs and spices:

- If you buy fresh herbs in bulk, you can freeze a certain amount and use them next time you're prepping food for the week

- Dare to experiment and make your own spice mix or herb mix, but make sure you don't use too many combinations

- When there is some unfamiliar herb or spice in a recipe (or herb/spice you don't use frequently) feel free to substitute it for an herb or spice you use often

- Use fresh herbs when you start cooking, while dried herbs should be added later. Also, herbs like sage, thyme, rosemary, oregano, etc. should be added in the early cooking process while delicate herbs such as tarragon, parsley, cilantro, chives and basil should be added at the last minute

- Don't season directly into the steaming pot as the steam could degrade the potency of spices or herbs left in the jar.

Experimenting with recipes

Meal prepping gives you the opportunity to try out new recipes and experiment with different meals; it's the variety that was already mentioned above. Below, you can see some tips that will help you decide what recipes to choose and how to organize them:

- Don't only opt for easy recipes; adjust the level of difficulty to the amount of time you have to prep them

- When trying new recipes, write down your reactions to it, e.g. enjoyed it, thinking about changing amounts to make it better, etc.

- Keep in mind number of servings. As you already know, portions are important for meal prep and number of servings allows you to adjust the ingredients amounts in case you need more or less servings

- Assume there will be leftovers and plan on what you will do with them.

How to easy-prep recipes using five main ingredients or less—this diet requires no costly or specialty foods

Ketogenic diets do not require you to eat expensive, specialist, or unusual food. That's one of the key benefits of this diet, that it's good wholesome food that is easy to get hold of, doesn't require lots of ingredients that you have to buy a large amount of to just use one tea-spoon then it's stuck in your cupboard until the expiry date has gone. Most of these ingredients, you'll already have in your house, or can get hold of from your nearest supermarket.

In this chapter, we'll look at how you can eat a ketogenic diet, and make meals out of 5 or 6 key ingredients.

5 Ingredient Ham and Cheese pockets
Ingredients:

85g of Ham

85 g of Mozarella (you can buy it ready grated, or else grate or chop into small pieces so that it's easier for it to melt).

85g of sliced cheese

1 large heaped tablespoon of cream cheese

4 tablespoons of flax seed meal

Method:

1. Melt the cream cheese and mozzarella in a bowl in the microwave (or if you don't have a microwave you can place a bowl over a pan of hot water, making sure no water enters the bowl itself, and melt the cheese this.
2. Add the flax meal to this, stir it in, to create dough.
3. Roll the dough out. In order to do this and create nice neat dough, you could place it between 2 bits of parchment (baking) paper, or you could use a silicone mat and silicone rolling pin.

4. In your dough that you've rolled out, place the ham and your sliced cheese.
5. Next fold the dough around this filling.
6. Finally, use a fork to poke some holes in the dough with the prongs, which will allow steam to release when the parcel is baking.
7. Bake it for 15-20 minutes at 200c, until browned.
8. Remove from oven, let it cool for a while, cut it in half and eat whilst it's still warm.

This recipe will take about 30 minutes in total. The ingredients make enough for 2 parcels.

Nutritional Details:

Per 1 parcel serving – Carbohydrates = 7.3g; Protein 32.5g; Fat = 31.3g (of that 15.4g is saturated).

2 Ingredient Banana Pancakes

Ingredients:

1 Large Banana

1 Large Egg

Method:

Peel a banana, and cut it into slices. Mash the banana using a fork, and combine the mashed banana with the egg. Mix this together until if fully combined into a batter.

Spray a frying pan with cooking spray (it's possible to buy 1 cal sprays). Heat the pan. Fill ¼ of a cup with the pancake batter and tip this into the frying pan.

Cook each side, until the pancake is lightly brown.

This recipe, should give you enough for 3 small pancakes. This is very inexpensive and therefore perfect if you're on a budget.

You could add a knob of butter onto the top of the pancake.

There's no flour involved at all in this recipe, which makes it idea. It's a quick and easy recipe to do. Very healthy. Smells and tastes great. If you're on a low carbohydrate diet, you could add a few berries over the top of your pancake also.

Nutritional Details: Per pancake: Carbohydrates 9g; Fat 1.5g; Sodium 24mg; Potassium 164 mg; Protein 2g; calories 58.

1 ingredient Mediterranean Pork Chops (plus seasoning)

Ingredients:

4 pork loin chops

½ tea spoon of Himalayan pink rock salt

¼ teaspoon of black pepper

1 tablespoon of fresh rosemary

2 garlic cloves

Method:

1. Sprinkle the salt and pepper over the chops.
2. 2. Next in a separate bowl crush/mince 2 cloves of garlic, and mix with the freshly chopped rosemary. Rub this over both sides of the pork chops.
3. Put the chops into an oven-proof roasting tin or dish. Cook for the first 10 minutes at 425; then turn the oven down to 350 and cook for a further 25 minutes.

Nutritional Details:

Per 1 pork chop: Fat – 4g; Carbohydrates – 1g; Fibre – 24g; Sodium – 288mg; Calories 147.

5 Ingredient Low-Carbohydrate Pizza

Ingredients:

¾ cup of mozzarella

½ cup of Marinara sauce

4 slices of pepperoni

½ tsp of basil

½ tsp of oregano

Method:

Put ½ of your mozzarella cheese into a frying pan, and allow it to heat and melt and it will caramelize too. When it's reasonably dark in colour, use a spatula to lift the disk of cheese from out of the frying pan. This will be the base for your pizza.

2. Next pour over the marina sauce making sure it covers all your cheese base and goes right to the edges.

3. Place the remaining mozzarella on top of the pizza, and the pepperoni slices too.

4. Sprinkle on the seasoning of basil and oregano.

5. Heat under a grill until the mozzarella on top of the pizza has melted.

Nutritional Details:

Fat – 29g; Carbohydrates – 6g; Protein – 24g; Calories 400g. This is for the entire pizza – this is 1 serving, if you eat the entire pizza as a meal.

5 Ingredient Breakfast muffins (Plus seasoning)

Ingredients:
6 eggs
1-2 small onions, finely chopped.
4-8 thin slices of chorizo, salami or cooked bacon.
1 tablespoon of red pesto
4 oz of grated cheese.
Seasoning (salt & pepper)

Method:
Preheat oven to 175.

Chop the onions and the bacon/chorizo/salami.

Whisk the eggs in a dish, add in the seasoning, and pesto, then stir in the cheese.

Pour the muffin batter into 12 of the muffin tray holes.

Bake in the oven for 15-20 minutes.

These can be eaten cold, and this makes them perfect for the whole family to take as a delicious savoury snack for packed lunches.

Nutritional Details:

Per serving of 1 muffin:

Fat:24.29g (of which 12.9g is saturated); Carbohydrates, 1.39g; Protein, 16.04g. Calories, 289.

5 Ingredient Strawberry Milkshake

Ingredients:
¼ cup of coconut milk or double-cream
¾ cup of almond milk
½ cup of strawberries
1 tablespoon of MCT oil or Extra Virgin Coconut Oil (MCT oil is better for you)
½ teaspoon of vanilla extract
It is possible to add stevia, if you'd like it to taste sweeter; you can also add 1 tablespoon of Chia seeds if you want this thicker and for more energy. If you add chia seeds, then I would either soak them the night before, or leave them in your milkshake throughout the day and drink the milkshake in the evening, so they have time to soften and swell

Method:
Mix the milk, and add the strawberries. Place these into a blender. Blend until smooth. Serve and Drink.

Nutritional Details:
These ingredients above make 1 serving. This serving contains: 27.4g of fat (of which 23.9 is saturated); 8.4g of carbs; 2g of fibre; 2.5g of protein; 35mg of magnesium; 234mg of potassium; 275 calories.

Simple yet delicious Keto recipes

Meat Pie

This pie looks stunning, and is tasty and can be served as part of an evening meal ideally at a lukewarm temperature; or you could slice it and take it cold for packed-lunch.

Ingredients for the filling:
1 finely chopped onion
1 finely chopped garlic clove
2 tablespoons of butter or olive oil
1 1/3 lbs of minced beef or lamb
Seasoning: salt and pepper
1 tbsp of dried oregano
4 tbsps of tomato puree
120ml of water

Ingredients for the pie-crust:
255g of almond flour
4 tbsp of sesame seeds
4 tbsp of coconut
1 tbsp of dried psyllium husk
1 tsp baking powder
A pinch of salt
3 tbsp of olive oil
1 egg
4 tbsp of water

Topping:
½ lb of cottage cheese
7 oz grated cheese

Method:
Pre-heat your oven to 75 degrees. In a frying pan, fry the onion, garlic and butter until soft. Add the minced meat, until it is browned. Add in oregano, salt and pepper. Next add the tomato puree. Add the water. Reduce the heat and just allow the ingredients to very gently bubble for 20 minutes.
Whilst that is gently bubbling, you can be getting on with the pie-crust.

For the pie crust the method couldn't be easier. Simply place all the ingredients into a food processor and mix them up until they form a call of dough.

Line a 10" oven proof pie-dish with grease-proof paper. Then place the pie-crust dough into the base and around the edges. Bake the pie crust for 10-15 minutes.

Fill the pie crust with the meat filling, place the cottage and grated cheese on top, then bake for a further 30 – 40 minutes.

Nutritional Details:
This meal is 70% fat; 25% protein, and 5% carbohydrates.

Size of Portions:
This pie gives 6 servings.

Chocolate Pots

Ingredients:

- 2 ½ large avocados – obviously peel the skin off and take out the centre stone. (Approx. 500g)
- ½ cup Cocoa powder (the higher the percentage of cocoa the better, aim for 70 -90% cocoa) (45g)
- 1 tsp of vanilla extract
- 2 tablespoons of extra virgin coconut oil
- pinch of pink Himalayan rock salt
- Some stevia as a natural sweetener. (usually ¾ od a teaspoon would be sufficient)
- 1-2 teaspoons of unsweetened almond *or* cashew milk
- Dark chocolate (ideally 70 – 90% cocoa content) – in order to make decorative curls on top of the pots.

Method:

1. This is a really simple technique. Place all the ingredients into a mixing bowl (with the exception of the dark chocolate, which is purely to make decorative curls on top of the pots) and mix with a hand blender until it's a smooth chocolate dessert consistency.
2. Pour into little glasses or ramekins and refrigerate.

3. Use a cold knife along the top of the bar of dark chocolate, or even a tablespoon edge, to create chocolate curls that you can place on the top of the chocolate pots.

Nutritional Details:

This is for per serving, so one chocolate pot; and the ingredients above make 4 servings.

Fat, 31.4g. Carbohydrate, 21.3 g. Fibre, 14.3g. Magnesium, 126 mg. Potassium, 887 mg. Calories – 337.

Chicken Casserole

Ingredients:

- 3 lbs chicken breasts or mini-fillets
- 1 tsp of pink Himalayan rock salt
- ½ tsp back pepper
- ¾ cup pesto (approx.. 7 oz) – it is possible to make your own pesto, especially if you grow basil in a herb garden/window box/plant pot in kitchen.
- 3 oz baby spinach (85 g)
- 300g of cherry tomatoes
- 400g of fresh mozzarella
- 50g of grated Parmesan cheese
- fresh basil to garnish

Method:

Preheat your oven to 200 degrees Celsius. Season the chicken with salt and pepper. Put half of the chicken into a casserole dish, and then place half of the pesto on to this.

Next, put half of the spinach on; and top this with half of the mozzarella.

Repeat with another layer.

Finally top the casserole with the parmesan cheese, and place the cherry tomatoes at the side of the dish.

Bake this in the oven for approximately 40-45 minutes, clearly until the chicken is properly cooked and white, and the cheese has melted and is slightly bubbling. You can place the dish under the grill, if you want to give your melted mozzarella a bit of a brown colouring. Place some fresh basil on the top of it before serving. This is a truly scrumptious dish, that is easy to do, but looks quite impressive. It's a meal that the entire family would enjoy.

Nutritional Details:

This recipe would serve 8 people. So, per serving, here are the nutritional values:

Fat, 28.9g (of which saturated is 8.7g). Carbohydrates, 4.6g. Fibre, 1.3g. Protein, 50.7g. Magnesium, 81mg. Potassium, 915 mg. Calories 486.

Paneer Curry

Ingredients:

- 200 g of paneer cheese
- 3 tbsp butter
- A bay leaf
- ½ tsp cumin seeds
- ½ large onion, chopped
- 2 medium tomatoes, chopped.
- 1 clove of garlic, chopped
- ½ inch of ginger, chopped
- ½ tsp turmeric powder
- ¼ tsp garam masala
- 80ml of double-cream
- fresh parsley for garnish
- Himalayan pink rock salt to season
- Fresh coriander
- ½ tbsp. of tomato paste
- You could decide to serve this with cauliflower rice. Cauliflower rice is just simply raw cauliflower that has been blitzed in a blender, to make it into rice size pieces, and boiled. It's a great low-carb alternative to rice.

Method:

1. Melt the butter in a saucepan, add in the bay leaf and the cumin seeds.

2. Next add the chopped onion, chopped garlic and the pinch of Himalayan pink rock salt. Cook on a low heat, until the onion is soft.
3. Add the tomatoes and tomato paste, fresh coriander, turmeric and ½ cup of water. Cook until the tomatoes have softened and are liquidy.
4. Remove the bay leaf and dispose of it. Put all of this into a blender, and blend until it is a smooth paste. If it appears too thick, you may add a little bit more water.
5. Cut the paneer into cubes (if it is not already cubed)
6. Put the paste back into a saucepan, and add the paneer cubes.
7. Let it simmer for 5 minutes.
8. Take the pan off the oven, and add the cream and garam masala.
9. Garnish with some fresh coriander and parsley.
10. You can serve this with cauliflower rice.

Nutritional Details:

Fat, 40.4g (of which 25.4g saturated). Carbohydrates, 10.2g. Fibre, 2.4g. Protein 15.6g. Magnesium, 16mg. Potassium 258mg. Calories 458.

Beef Spare Ribs

Ingredients:

- 8 spare beef ribs, approximately 2-3 lbs.
- 30g coconut oil
- 30g of ghee
- Pink Himalayan rock salt & pepper, to season
- ½ - 1 cup Marsala wine (or you can use dry white wine)
- 180ml of tomato puree
- 225g of tomatoes – cut up into chunks.
- 3 cloves chopped garlic
- 450g of cups cooked spinach
- 2 sticks of celery chopped
- 2 carrots
- 5 *mushrooms sliced.*

Method:

1. Cut the ribs into 8 even pieces. Season them with pink Himalayan rock salt and black pepper.
2. Pre-heat a frying pan, and place in the coconut oil and ghee.
3. Seal the ribs on all sides, ensuring they're brown.
4. Remove the ribs and place into a slow cooker.

5. Add the Marsala wine to the slow cooker, and all of the remaining ingredients. Ensure that everything has been given a good stir to ensure there are vegetables and sauce in all parts of the slow cooker pot.
6. Depending on a low heat for 8 hours. You shouldn't need to lift the lid, but if you do, just once, turn the ribs over.

This recipe looks and smells divine; it's a beautiful orangey/reddy colour. This recipe using the above amount of ingredients makes 4 servings.

Nutritional Details:

Fat: 39.9g (of which 21.4g are saturated). Carbohydrates, 8.7g. Fibre, 2.7g. Protein, 26.3g. Magnesium, 82mg. Potassium, 985mg. Calories, 512.

Bacon Wrapped & Cheese Stuffed Burgers

Ingredients:

Burgers:

- 2.5lbs of ground beef
- Pink Himalayan rock salt & pepper for seasoning
- 150g of thin-cut slices bacon
- 150g of grated cheddar cheese
- BBQ sauce
- Dijon mustard

Filling:

- 2 tbsp of <u>ghee</u>
- 1 medium onion, cut into slices.
- 250g of sliced peppers.
- 140g of sliced mushrooms.

Method:

1. Place ghee into a frying pan, and melt. Then add the sliced onion and cook until the onion is softened and just starting to brown.
2. Add the sliced peppers, it can be a nice idea to use differing colours here, to give your meal a nice vibrant feel. If it looks colourful and

appetizing, you'll enjoy eating it more. So, you could use, yellow, orange and red peppers.
3. Add the mushrooms and cook all this for a further 3-5 minutes.
4. Take the ground beef and make into 6 burgers. To make sure they're of an even size you can half the mixture, half again, and half again.
5. Flatten each burger, so that it looks typically burger shaped, then take a very small glass and use it to press into the centre of the burger, so that you're essentially creating an indentation, a little bit of well for the filling, like a bowl, or a very small pencil holder/vase.
6. Wrap 2 slices of the bacon around the outside of your miniature vase and remove the glass.
7. Fill the centre of each meat bowl with the onion, peppers and some Dijon mustard.
8. Finally, top this with grated cheese. Do the same for all the other burgers.
9. Once all your burgers have been shaped and created. Place them on a tray in the oven on 150 degrees Celsius, and cook for 45 – 60 minutes. When they're cooked, remove from the oven, and let them cool for 5 minutes, before eating.
10. You could serve with some salad, or green low-carbohydrate vegetables.

Nutritional Details:

The ingredients above will make 6 burgers. The details below are for 1 serving of 1 burger.

Fat: 60.6g (of which 26.5g are saturated); Carbohydrates, 6.6 g. Fibre, 1.9g. Protein, 46.g. Magnesium, 60mg. Potassium 88- mg. Calories, 767.

Ketogenic Diet as a Permanent Lifestyle Change

One of the key premises of this diet is that eat good healthy food. This is saying in a nutshell is that the Ketogenic diet is NOT a 'diet' that is going to limit your portion size. It's NOT a diet whereby you eat a meal and then are ravenously hungry five minutes later. It's about making a lifestyle change, whereby you make Ketogenic choices and decisions about the food you eat, and eat more fat, and less carbohydrate, and therefore feel full and satisfied and interested and excited by the food you eat. A Ketogenic diet fully acknowledges that dieting is only a small part of what will become a lifestyle change for you. The whole concept of a Ketogenic diet is that there's much more to you becoming happy and successful, than just watching the weighing scales each week. This diet book, also takes into account your emotions and wants you to keep track of how you feel, especially your levels of happiness. The diet also seeks to work on your levels of confidence too and really to give these a boost. This book wants people who follow a Ketogenic diet to be happy, content, confident, healthier and to feel satisfied that they've eaten enough food, and also do not have a limited diet. On this diet, clearly Carbohydrates are limited and restricted; but we hope to show you, that a Ketogenic diet is exciting, and there are lots of alternatives you can have to carbohydrates. For example, if you're wanting alternatives to rice, try cauliflower rice. If you want alternatives to spaghetti, try 'courgetti spaghetti' which are courgettes that have been spiralized. Or sweet potato works too ... but do watch the carbohydrate levels with this, and only have this occasionally.

If you have Type 2 Diabetes; or are under the age of 16 years old; are a nursing mum; or if you're going through the menopause. If you fit into any of these categories, it is always worth speaking with both your Doctor, before embarking on a Ketogenic diet. It could be that for diabetics, this diet is perfect for you and will naturally lower your blood sugar and the need for insulin. But, you'll need the help of a Dr, to ensure that everything is at the correct level that it should be. If you're a nursing Mum do speak to you Doctor or Health Visitor. Using a Ketogenic diet can help with Type 2 Diabetes to offer a healthy living approach, but do speak with your diabetic health care professional before starting the diet. Using a ketogenic diet throughout the menopause should help ease menopausal symptoms, but again check with your Doctor before starting. The Ketogenic diet is not suitable for you if you have a diagnosis of bulimia nervosa or anorexia nervosa because this usually means that you lose more weight.

In this book, you will learn the difference between the different types of cholesterol. You'll learn about what foods you can and can't eat. You'll learn how you can eat additional carbohydrates if you exercise more. You'll learn what the sensible amount of weight you should be losing per week; you'll learn about foods which it is better for you to eat; you'll learn about super foods and what these do to your body and mind; you'll become familiar with the; you' concept of ketosis, you'll have seen a meal plan and various ketogenic recipes above.

People who are serious about embarking on a Ketogenic diet, know it's not just a fad diet, and not a diet that is a 'crash-course' in losing weight fast, but instead, more about a lifestyle change, where you eat healthier, feel better, change your metabolism for the better and this is something that is manageable for the duration, because it's about eating good, healthy, tasty meals and being supported to do so. Whilst carbohydrates are restricted, the rest of the diet is enormously flexible and focuses around good wholesome food. It's a diet that fits around people's real lives. It's personalised and tailored to individuals. There are different ketogenic diets you can follow but this book focusses mostly on the standard Ketogenic diet.

There has been evidence to support that people lose more weight by following a Ketogenic diet, than by following a low fat diet.

You may decide that a strict low carbohydrate diet, of eating just 5% of carbohydrates isn't practical for you. If you decide this, you could just go for a reduced carbohydrate diet, but do be aware, that if you choose to do this, it may take you longer to reach that desired state of Ketosis.

When you decide to follow a Ketogenic diet, especially at first until you get fully into the swing of it, it can be a really good idea to keep track of what food, and what quantities of food you're consuming. I would use a notebook, or an online tracker, or create some sort of table for yourself. This way, you can measure exactly what you're eating.

Another key reason for tracking things to, is to consider your emotional state, and ability to think clearly. A Later chapter called in this book called Positivity is the part of this Ketogenic lifestyle change that deals with your emotions, motivation and positivity. It's a way of making sure your mental health is supporting you to be where you need to be to diet physically. It's about boosting your self-confidence and learning to love yourself once again.

This is part of the holistic approach of this book that looks at the whole person and realises that it's about the whole person in order for weight changes to be a success.

How fast can you lose weight?

The recommended amount for people to lose per week, and manage to keep that weight-loss off, is 1-2lbs per week. Most dieters who have a lot to lose, would in truth like to lose more than that, because it's natural that they want to see quick results. But, the best approach is one which is slow and steady, 1-2lbs per week. By losing this amount, you WILL keep the weight loss off, much better than if you were to go on a crash-diet, or extreme diet which can often be based on shakes/soups and little else. That type of diet, is not sustainable long-term! No-one wants to live on liquid shakes and soups for the rest of their lives. Food would become very boring indeed, and everything is liquefied, there's not texture or crunch. The second that you resume a normal diet, after a crash or extreme diet, the weight will balloon again, and people often become heavier than when they initially started to diet.

If you have a lot of weight to lose; you may find that in your very first week of dieting, you do lose more than 1-2 lbs per week, and this is Ok and not dangerous. But, you will also find, that after a few weeks of losing bigger amounts, your weight loss will level off, and become 1-2lbs per week, and this is fine. Don't be disappointed by this. Every single pound, or even half a pound, is weight off, and closer towards your target weight. Every week that you eat more healthily will do wonders for your overall physical and mental health. Do remember that many of your body's organs rejuvenate themselves over time. The more you can put good food into your body, with fresh fruit and veg and lots of healthy vitamins, the healthier all your organs will become. This diet too is about avoiding carbohydrates and eating more fat too.

If you haven't lost weight in a week, then there are a few areas you can check to ensure you haven't fallen into a pitfall. Consider whether your food portion size have been creeping up? It can be worth re-measuring bowls of cereal, and putting a limit on the milk you drink in tea/coffee. Are you accounting for sauces/gravy? Have you definitely been tracking all the food you've consumed, and have not had any naughty snacks here and there? Have you eaten out more? Are you eating an excessive amount carbohydrates for this Ketogenic diet, beyond the point of fulfilling your hunger, to becoming stuffed? Have you been drinking alcohol? As sometimes this can take you out of ketosis.

Some people who have issues with digesting meat, and feel sluggish and lethargic after eating it, sometime opt to eat more of a Mediterranean diet, this type of diet includes salads, lots of tomatoes, fruit, garlic, vegetable-pasta, sauce, soups, olives and olive oils are good, things like hummus with vegetable crudités to dip in, can be good. Eggs are good, you could make vegetable frittatas. Add herbs and spices. Mediterranean diets can often tend to follow seasonal produce, so depending on the time of year, depends on whether it is spring, summer, autumn or winter vegetables that will be more readily available and used. You can opt to eat more cheese and fish, it doesn't have to be so meat orientated.

Another reason for not losing weight could be that you have water retention which will make you weigh heavier, and could be the cause of tight feeling skin on your calves, or around your ankles, or a bloated stomach, or fingers that feel swollen and tight. If you think you have water retention and don't have any other known medical conditions or anything impairing your kidneys, then you could try buying some Boldo & Herb tablets from a Health Food shop, or some Dandelion coffee or tablets because these act as a diuretic; another option which may seem counter-intuitive is to drink more water – please see the chapter on water later in this book, for more details as to why drinking water prevents water retention. If you have any health conditions though, please consult your Doctor first to see if it is suitable for you to take them. Yoghurts and cottage cheese are good. The yoghurt can provide excellent bacteria which is needed for good digestive health. It's really beneficial to ensure your yoghurts are sugar-free; and things like probiotics in yoghurts can be good.

Gadgets

There are a few kitchen gadgets that may help the weight to fall off that bit quicker. Having a good quality non-stick rolling pins and chopping boards means that when you're making non-carb pastry, whatever you use will not become all sticky and stick to the rolling pin. Having some kitchen scales, will allow you to keep track of portion sizes. You don't have to weigh out your food every time once you have a good idea of what size a portion is, say for example of butter, or cauli-flower rice. But, every now and then it is worth re-weighing your portions, just to check that over time, you're not being overly generous with them. Because ultimately, you're only fooling yourself and the weight will take longer to come off. Having lots of food storage containers, and food-bags can be really effective. You don't have to purchase expensive Tupperware ones, you can pick up plastic box containers, or tin-foil take-out style boxes from Pound/Dollar Stores. Having soup bags can be an excellent way of making a large batch of soup, having a bowl and freezing the rest in soup-bags for whenever you fancy some. By having plenty of food containers, this means that you can cook in batch too. So, if you make a lot of curry or chili or Shepherd's pie for example, and wish to freeze some for a meal another evening, you have the option to do so. Finally, another gadget which can help when you're dieting is a Julienne peeler, or spiralizer – both do a very similar thing, they enable you to get fine strands of vegetable, such as courgettes or sweet potatoes, so that they look similar to spaghetti. Sweet potato spaghetti with meat balls, can make a truly delicious dish.

What is worth remembering is that weight was gained over months/years. It will take months/years to come off, depending on how much weight you have to lose. Be prepared to be in this for the long haul, and ultimately, for life. If you're expecting to shed all the weight you want to lose in a couple of weeks, you'll be disappointed. But, do take each pound or even half pound you lose as a step towards your overall weight-loss goal. Any weight off, is better than on. Also if you lose 2lbs (regardless of how many weeks it takes you to do that) celebrate that as a momentous achievement! 2lbs is the weight of a bag of sugar, or a bag of flour. Now, as silly as this may seem, if I told you to walk around with a bag of flour hanging off the end of your nose all day ... or even to carry a bag of flour around with you all day. That will soon get VERY heavy, and

VERY tiresome to carry around. That weight is no longer on your body!

Body mass index

The Body Mass Index (BMI) is calculated by a person's mass, ie how much they weigh, divided by the square of the body height. BMI is usually worked out by taking into account weight in kilogrammes and height in metres. Often you'll find BMI tables/graphs that give you an indication of what your optimum weight 'should' be, for the height that you are. The BMI attempts to take into account in your weight, your muscle, fat and bone, and then will determine if you're underweight, normal, overweight or classed in the obese category. For adults if their BMI falls under 18.5 they may be classed as underweight. Normal BMI weight is between 18.5 – 25. Overweight is categorised as 25 – 30, and if you have a BMI that is over 30 that's classed as obese. If someone has a BMI under 15 they are very severely underweight and malnourished and classed as starving. If someone has a BMI of less than 17.5, this is usually classed as anorexia nervosa. The obesity section falls into three categories. 30-35 is class 1, moderately obese. 35-40 is class 2 severely obese. And 40 + is class three, very severely obese.

If you're into the overweight and obese ranges, then there can be a much greater risk of contracting heart-disease, strokes and Type II diabetes.

BMI can be used as a 'general' guide, but doesn't always work perfectly for individuals, especially if people are very tall, or very short. It doesn't always take into account the type of frame that a person has either. There are other exceptions to the BMI index, which includes children, the elderly, the infirm and athletes. The BMI doesn't distinguish between muscle mass, and fat mass either.

Some countries set different guidelines as to BMI, Hong Kong for example, classes a BMI of 23 – 25 as overweight, and anything from 25 upwards as obese. Japan also have obesity as starting at a BMI of 25. Singapore also has their BMI of obesity as being a BMI of 23 or more, and state that if your BMI is over 23, you're at moderate risk of developing heart disease, high blood pressure, stroke and diabetes, and if your BMI is over 27.5, then you're at high risk of developing those.

With America in particular the population of both men and women over 60% of the population is overweight or obese. The World Health Organisation (WHO) use the BMI index to measure obesity. Some countries such as France, Spain, Italy and Israel use the BMI to put legislation in place for models, and will not allow people to have a BMI of less than 18, in order to fight anorexia amongst models.

One of the key things to take into account with the Body Mass Index (BMI) is that it's a rough estimate of what your ideal body weight should be. It's not 100% accurate. It's not set in stone. If you reach a weight, that is higher than what your BMI suggests, and you're personally happy with that, and feel comfortable, that's fine! If you head towards your BMI and if for any reason your friends/family members start to comment that you're looking 'thin' or 'unhealthy' or 'gaunt' then you may wish to readjust your weight goals, and consider the BMI as too low in weight for you and set your own target that you feel healthy at.

You will be able to find BMI calculators online, where you can check what your BMI is estimated to be; some weighing scales you can purchase too give this information to you.

By losing 10% of your body weight, this can have immense health benefits. It will immediately lower your cholesterol, and reduce your blood pressure. Both of these factors being high, put you at far greater risk of heart disease. By losing 10% of your body weight, it will mean that you'll improve the chances of your body being able to use the insulin it produces. If your body can't do this, then you're more at risk of developing Type II Diabetes. By losing 10% of your body weight, you'll feel a dramatic increase in how energetic your feel. You'll be able to walk without getting so out of breath. You'll be able to run easier. You'll feel more mentally alert. Knowing that you've managed to lose 10% of your body weight will give you a massive boost of self-confidence in your own will-power and this will be hugely motivational, to encourage you to keep on striving towards your weight goals. You will KNOW that you're capable of doing it, and being successful. You'll be able to assess once you've lost 10% whether you have the commitment to keep on losing more to reach your goal. Regardless, a 10% weight loss is absolutely incredible, and you deserve to be very proud and congratulate yourself.

Super foods

Super foods are foods that are super healthy for you to eat; they can often be foods that prevent illnesses, replace a deficiency or fight against obesity. Super foods are often known as whole-foods and can include foods such as Quinoa, Edamame Soybeans, and lentils; usually foods that are low in fat. Many super foods purport to reduce the risk of chronic diseases, that can include: cancer, stroke, heart-disease and diabetes. Superfoods are meant to rejuvenate you and slow down ageing, boost your immune system, prevent depression, and make people's minds more active. Some super foods are known as such, for the antioxidants they contain and omega-3 fatty acids. Anti-oxidants can include beta-carotene (found in carrots), plus vitamins A, C and E, flavonoids and selenium (good for strong hair and nails). Cells in your body are attacked by free radicals that cause damage; antioxidants protect cells against free radicals.

So, to specify some food which it's good to try and incorporate into your diet, you could consider the following:

Garlic is very good for lowering people's cholesterol and blood pressure which makes it good to combat heart-disease, it's also effective to boost the immune system and prevent colds/flu symptoms. Finally garlic is suppose to prevent some types of cancer too (especially bowel and stomach cancer, and may assist with ovarian, colon and prostate cancer). Garlic contains vitamins B6 and C, manganese, selenium, and allicin. Garlic clearly has a very distinctive flavour and aroma and can really add a lot to different recipes.

Blueberries contain vitamin C, fibre, Vitamin K, manganese and anthocyanins. Blueberries are purported to prevent heart-disease by up to a third (if three portions of blueberries are consumed per week), preventing cancer and be good for boosting your memory. Blueberries may prevent atherosclerosis (the hardening of the arteries responsible for causing heart-attacks and strokes). Blueberries can lower blood pressure. Blueberries can prevent free-radical damage to cells. Blueberries can easily be added to breakfast cereals or porridge, or you can put them in a pot with packed lunch to nibble on, place them in flap-jack bars, add them to fruit smoothies, or to a yoghurt to make it more snazzy.

Goji berries seem to be one of the latest super food crazes to be pushed by health food shops and online retailers. They have been used in Chinese herbal medicine for years. They're often connected to various celebrities and purported to boost the brain, immune system, give you longevity, and protect against disease. Goji berries do indeed contain a good source of vitamins, including A, C, B2, selenium, iron, and polysaccharides. It has been reported that drinking Goji berry juice can make people feel good, have good digestion and increase brain activity.

Beetroot contains iron and folic acid. It also contains magnesium, nitrates, betaine and betacyanin. Beetroot purports to be able to lower blood pressure due to it containing nitric oxide, prevent dementia by increasing blood-flow to the brain; and help people perform better when participating in exercise or sports if they've been drinking beetroot juice.

Green Tea has long been used by Chinese herbalists because the leaves have strong antioxidants in them. Green tea also includes B Vitamins, folic acid, magnesium, potassium and catechins. Green tea is purported to prevent cancer (especially effective with stomach and breast cancer), and Alzheimer's disease (by protecting nerve cells from dying, which occurs in Alzheimer's), reduce heart-disease, lower cholesterol due to its catechins; reduce blood pressure thus lowering the risk of heart-disease and strokes; and to help weight loss by speeding up the metabolism and thus burning more calories. Green tea can also be used as an effective mouth wash that prevents tooth-decay.

Pomegranate Juice contains vitamins A, C, E, iron and tannins. It's a beautiful jewel like fruit, which is perfect in drinks, or its seeds add vibrancy, crunch and flavour to salads. Pomegranates are purported to be effective at lowering high blood pressure, relieving inflammation, offering protection against cancer (especially prostate by drinking 8oz of pomegranate juice per day) and reducing the risk of heart disease (it reduces cholesterol build up in arteries and increases blood flow to the heart). Pomegranate can be used to strengthen bones and reduce osteoporosis. It is REALLY important to note that if you're buying pomegranate juice from a supermarket, to ensure that in the ingredients you are getting 100% pomegranate juice, and that it's not a carton or bottle that contains added sugar.

Broccoli comes in your regular green variety, but also a purple sprouting form too. Broccoli contains Vitamins A, C and K, folic acid, beta-carotene, calcium, fibre, sulforaphane and indole-3-carbinol. Broccoli is purported to reduce the risk of cancer (especially mouth, throat and stomach cancer). The sulforaphane in broccoli can prevent damage to small blood vessels caused by high blood sugar (as in the case of diabetes). Broccoli is a cruciferous vegetable, which can help protect against free radical damage. You can use broccoli as an accompanying vegetable to a main meal, in stir-fries, soups, and curries. You need to eat 80g of broccoli to count towards one of the ten-a-day portions of fruit and vegetables that you should be ideally consuming.

Oily Fish contains vitamins B, D, selenium, protein and is a good source of omega-3 fatty acids, which has excellent health benefits. Oily fish include fish such as salmon, mackerel and sardines. Oily fish is purported to fight cardiovascular disease by lowering blood pressure, and reducing the chance of fat building up in arteries; it can reduce the risk of contracting cancer (especially prostate); it can prevent the loss of vision due to age, and dementia. The UK government recommends that people eat 2 portions of fish per week, one of these should be oily fish. If people eat two or more portions of oily fish per week, this has been proven to demonstrate the prevention of eye deterioration. Studies have also shown that if women eat one portion of oily fish per week, they're a third less likely to develop rheumatoid arthritis than those who did not eat it. Part of the rationale behind recommending people eat oily fish, was due to the fact that the Eskimo population whose diet largely consists of oily fish, have far fewer heart attacks and strokes. Food items like tinned sardines and mackerel are cheap, easy to keep in your food cupboards, and very easy to have on toast or with a side-salad as a healthy meal.

Chocolate – my guess, is that if you're anything like me, and you're reading a diet book, and see 'chocolate' listed as a super-food, that's the first food in the list I would turn to read about. Chocolate?!? Sounds like heaven, right? There are Kuna Indians in Panama who regularly drink cocoa as their main drink, and this group of people had low blood pressure, which meant they were less at risk of contracting heart-attacks and strokes. Cocoa itself contains magnesium, zinc, iron, catechins and procyanidins, manganese and phosphorous. It's when that goes through the process of turning it into chocolate, that sweeteners, fat and milk are added (which clearly can lead to weight gain). However, dark chocolate in particular, has many of the health benefits of cocoa. You can buy dark chocolate which has various percentages of cocoa, and obviously the higher the cocoa the better the chocolate is for you. Dark chocolate purports to protect against cancer, and to lower stress levels in the body. Studies have shown that dark chocolate can lower blood pressure, thus improving cardiovascular health, another study has shown that people who eat chocolate are less likely to have a stroke than those who never eat it.

Flavonoids, found in dark chocolate (and red wine) may help to ease leg/foot ulcers.

Wheatgrass contains vitamins A, C and E, calcium, magnesium, iron and chlorophyll. Wheatgrass is purported to reduce inflammation (which can be particularly good if you have something like ulcerative colitis (inflammation of the colon), increase your red blood cells, and as a result improve your circulation. Studies have looked at patients with Thalassaemia (a blood disorder) and when they drank wheatgrass juice each day, they required far fewer blood transfusions. You could put some wheatgrass juice into a smoothie of other fruit and vegetables, to give your body an added boost.

Quinoa (pronounced 'keen-wah') is a high protein grain, by eating it, it enables the body to build protein. Quinoa is good for preventing diabetes by lowering blood sugar when eaten. Quinoa is also beneficial for lowering hypertension. One very beneficial aspect to Quinoa is that it's purported to work as an appetite suppressant, making you less hungry and less likely to want to binge eat other food that is higher in carbohydrates. Because it's high in protein and low in calories, it makes it an ideal healthy food source. Quinoa contains phenols, which help to destroy free radicals, and thus slows down ageing process, and reduces the risk of contracting cancer. Quinoa is gluten free which makes it a great grain, for those with gluten intolerance; many more people have not yet realised they're intolerant to wheat and gluten, and when they reduce this in their diet, they can notice a big weight-loss. Quinoa contains riboflavin, which can really help migraine sufferers; it also contains saponins which help skin to heal from injury.

Edamame Soybeans feature as part of Asian cuisine. They're green beans in their pods (or they may have been popped) that have a slightly sweet taste because they're young and soft. They contain fibre, protein and lots of anti-oxidants. They're considered to be a very healthy food for dieters. The beans are a perfect accompaniment to means, but you can also create hummus with it, or pesto, or use in a stir-fry dish as a great source of protein. Edamame is a good source of protein (and the plant protein rather than animal protein lowers cholesterol, which reduces hardening of the arteries, that can lead to heart-attacks and strokes). Edamame also contains iron, magnesium and calcium (so can be beneficial if people suffer from migraines). Eating Edamame can reduce the risk of heart-attacks and diabetes. Edamame contains isoflavones which can reduce the risk of osteoporosis. The more soy people consume, the less likelihood there is of getting dementia and

Alzheimer's. Soybeans contain Genistein which is an antioxidant that prevents against free radical damage, and it's been found that if women eat 10mg of soy per day, this makes them 25% less likely to get breast cancer. It contains natural folic acid, which can give you a mood boost, by preventing the build-up of homocysteine in the body; when this builds up, the hormones that make you feel good such as serotonin, dopamine and norepinephrine can't get through and this impacts upon how you feel, your sleep pattern, and can make you more likely to binge or comfort eat. The folic acid can also be highly beneficial if you're planning on starting a family to help with fertility. The iron in the Edamame will give you more energy. Finally, the choline in Edamame reduces inflammation.

Lentils are a great superfood, they're very high in protein (they contain more protein than beef), you can buy great big bags of them relatively cheaply which can make them a good food source if you're on a budget, and they're really versatile to use in a range of dishes, that are also ideal for vegetarians and vegans. Lentils contain folic acid, potassium, iron (which can be excellent to prevent anaemia, and give you an energy boost) and antioxidants. Lentils are very good to reduce inflammation. Lentils contain fantastic fibre (one serving has three times the fibre of a bowl of bran flakes!) which is excellent at reducing cholesterol, thus helping to reduce the risk of heart disease. Often we tend to think that raw or gently cooked food is better at retaining nutrients and vitamins, but our bodies absorb the calcium, zinc and iron from lentils easily once they're cooked. There's a wide range of recipes that utilize lentils, including peppers stuffed with lentils and goats cheese; there's a wonderful red lentil and aubergine curry that is delicious.

Water for Weight Loss

One of the key things you can do to increase your chances of weight loss, are to drink as much water as you possibly can; up to eight glasses a day. If you can manage to drink 3 litres a day that is the optimum amount, but two litres would be good if that's all you can manage. If you build drinking water into your daily routine, it will become common-place and habitual. Eight glasses of water may sound a lot. But, if the second you wake up you drink a glass of water. If you drink a glass of water when you arrive at work, have one in your break at 11am. Have a glass of water at lunch time. One in your afternoon break at 3pm. Have a glass of water as soon as you get home from work. One throughout the evening, and one just before you go to bed, that would be your eight glasses of water a day, spread throughout the day and evening and is quite manageable and achievable. There are so many benefits about drinking water, that it could fill an entire book on its own. However, keeping it brief, the water will flush out any toxins, it will make your skin glow, eyes look brighter and less baggy with dark circles under them, your skin will become hydrated and will plump out in a healthy way making wrinkles disappear and skin less dull, grey and saggy, it'll instead look rejuvenated and young.

Your skin is a barrier that prevents fluid loss from your body, so it makes sense that if you're dehydrated, this barrier is going to look dry and wrinkled, whilst you can apply moisturiser to the outer surface of your skin, it needs to be hydrated from the inside too. Water will greatly aid digestion, and make all food flow through your body more efficiently. When you're dehydrated, your body can't flush out toxins and these cause disease and sickness, premature ageing, and weight gain.

Drinking water will boost your metabolism, meaning that you'll burn calories more quickly. Drinking water will get rid of any waste products in your body. Drinking water before every main meal or snack-time as suggested in the above paragraph, will also serve to work as an appetite suppressant, by filling your body up with water, it'll mean you're less hungry and less prone to binge eat or over-eat. It can make you feel fuller, and research has proven that by doing this you're likely to eat 75 calories less per meal, that would soon add up over a day, and over a week the results would be dramatic.

Studies have shown that people who upped their water intake, but didn't change anything else in the lifestyle, lost weight over a year, in comparison to those who did not up their water intake. Now, clearly we're suggesting here that you up your water intake, and follow the Ketogenic diet to achieve good effects, but this is proof of the benefits that drinking water has.

If you're a person who drinks a lot of fizzy drinks, these are full of sugar, ad high in calorie value; by replacing these drinks with bottled water, this would be so much healthier for you. Also, fizzy drinks can often contain the artificial sweetener aspartame which can impact seriously and detrimentally on your health. Water doesn't contain this. Even fruit juice is quite high in sugar naturally, so water is better for you than this.

If you find water a little plain to taste, there are so many fruit diffuser bottles now on the market that have a centre core with holes in, which allow the flavours of the natural fruit to diffuse into your water. You could add lemon and lime, or apple, or berries, to give your water a fruity taste. You could add cucumber to make your water really refreshing; or mint leaves. Apparently if the water you drink is ice-cold, then your body has to work harder to bring this up to body temperature, so this will boost your metabolism. You don't have to buy a special diffuser bottle, you could simply decide to keep a jug of water in the fridge (or a bowl/saucepan/any container) and place some lime/lemon into it, and top up your glass or water bottle using this. Losing weight does not have to be expensive. Diffusing some ginger root in the water, is a really nice taste, and it's also a great anti-emetic, good if you're feeling a bit nauseous, perhaps after a night out.

The effect of drinking water on your body, will mean that you're far less likely to suffer from muscle cramps and achey joints. Being properly hydrated will make your body much more likely to be able to cope with exercise. Being hydrated will prevent your tummy from feeling bloated, sluggish and clogged up. Drinking water will also keep your teeth healthy and your mouth fresh, which will lessen the chance of halitosis.

One easy way to check how hydrated you are, is to check the colour of your urine when you go to the toilet. If your urine is dark yellow/orange, then this could be a sign that you're dehydrated (or have too much vitamin C in your body if you're taking vitamin C tablets). If your urine is a very clear, pale colour, then this is a sign that you're better hydrated. If you're hot either through exercise or the weather, drinking water will help to regulate your body temperature.

If you think you'll drink your water via drinking tea, then ensure your tea is decaffeinated, or ideally green tea, which is rich in anti-oxidants. There is a green tea diet, which recommends you drink 4 cups of green tea per day before meals. Again, if you combined green tea drinking with the Ketogenic diet, this can only be beneficial. It is worth knowing that green tea can dehydrate you, so you do need to keep drinking water in between the green tea.

It is possible to download apps that can help you to keep track of how much water you have drank. There are apps called 'Waterlogged' and 'Water Drink Reminder.' You could also decide to track this yourself on a note-book, or a table that you make. Or with an online app, where you can track what you eat and drink, so you could put how many bottles or glasses of water you have drank on there! My Fitness Pal is one such app you could decide to use. If you don't want to invest in a particular app, then you could simply set an alarm reminder on your mobile, or Outlook email, to remind you to drink more at certain points throughout the day.

When you start to feel thirsty, it's already too late really. You're already dehydrated by that point that your brain sends you the signal you're thirsty. At that stage, you've already lost 2% of your body's water. Given the fact that our bodies are made up of so much water, this is a significant amount for us. If you're exercising and dehydrated, your exercising won't be so effective.

Other research has shown that sometimes people confuse feeling hungry, with actually being thirsty. It's been shown too, that even when you eat something it can take 20 minutes for your brain to register that you're actually full and satisfied now.

So, you could try drinking a glass of water the next time you feel hungry, and waiting 20 minutes to see if you're genuinely hungry or just thirsty. If your stomach gurgles, you feel light-headed, or you feel low on energy, all of these symptoms could relate to being dehydrated.

Brains are mostly water, so it makes sense than when you're dehydrated, this will have a negative impact on the brain. It'll make you feel more anxious, have difficulty remembering things, it'll impact on your ability to concentrate. Drinking a decent amount of water will prevent headaches and migraines. If you drink water this will prevent constipation and instead have food flowing through your body with ease.

By drinking water, this will give you so much more energy. Because our bodies are 70% water, keeping this water topped up, will mean that your cells work as they should, your muscles will have oxygen and other vital nutrients, and your brain will be active and clear. If you're ever feeling tired or lethargic, then drink some water and this will give you a boost. Drinking water can boost your mental state putting you in a better mood, it can help you to concentrate and get rid of headaches. It is so good for all your body organs, and drinking decent amounts of water daily can prevent so many different diseases. When you drink water, your body makes no distinction between water and food, it will start to metabolize (burn the calories) of whatever you put into it. When you drink water your body will start to metabolize fat, which is done by the liver. The liver works closely with the kidneys, and these definitely need plenty of water to work effectively to flush out toxins. If your kidneys aren't working properly then your liver will try to do some of the work that your kidneys would normally have done, which then slows down the job of your liver in metabolizing fat. By keeping your kidneys flushed, this will prevent the build-up of mineral deposits, and will prevent things like kidney stones forming. If you haven't been kind to your kidneys and have consumed too much alcohol or salt, then be kind to them and give them a really good flush by drinking lots of water.

There's everything to gain and nothing to lose by doing this. Also, unlike other drinks you'd purchase, water is virtually free! You're paying your water bill each month or quarter anyhow, so why not make the most of it. If for any reason your tap water doesn't taste as nice as you'd like it to, then you're able to invest in a relatively inexpensive water filter.

Drinking water has been proved, time and time again, to reduce weight, and keep the weight off. It makes good sense to combine drinking water with the Ketogenic diet, and it will help you to avoid any less positive symptoms of the Ketogenic diet.

When you first start drinking more water, you will need to nip to the loo more frequently. But adding fresh water to your body, will mean that some of the old water your body has stored (as water retention) can be got rid of. It seems counter-intuitive sometimes that to get rid of water retention you need to drink more water, but, honestly that's how it works. Get rid of the old, and replace with new. Incidentally after a while of building up good water drinking habits, your body does become used to it, and the frequent need to urinate will happen less. Also your body will have less water retention as your body and mind will realise that you have this regular supply of water coming in, so there's no need to store (retain) as much water around your body. Avoid adding salt to food, as salt makes you retain water, in order to break the salt down and deal with it in your body. Most food you buy already has salt in it, so don't add any more. If you want a bit of seasoning, use pepper, or other herbs and spices.

If you like to have an alcoholic drink. A good tactic can be to match any alcohol you drink, with equal amounts of water. So, if you have a glass of wine, ensure you've drank a wine-glass full of water too. If you have a pint of beer, ensure that you've drank a pint of water.

Exercise

Part of a Ketogenic lifestyle is about getting you to move more. By moving more, you'll burn more calories and therefore will lose more weight, tone up, be healthier and will be in better shape. A Ketogenic lifestyle, is a full lifestyle change that encompasses the whole person. Therefore, you can't 'just' concentrate on cutting down what you eat, and tracking that. If you just did that, yes, you'd probably lose weight, but there's so much more to the Ketogenic way of life. It's all about taking a holistic approach, where you eat healthy choices, be the best person that you can be, have more energy, become less stressed, and move more (ie. Exercise).

Exercise helps you lose weight and become healthier; it also gives you more energy and produces endorphins that improve your mental state and put you in a good mood. Following a Ketogenic diet should not be onerous, and should be achievable and fun, we're not suggesting you necessarily set aside great periods of time per day to exercise, but simply make the best of the time you have available, and fit things into your daily routine where you can. Even 5 minutes here and there all add up ad can produce good results when you do it consistently. On a Ketogenic diet, it can be good to try to do 20-30 mins of resistance training 5 days a week, and take a more leisurely exercise approach for the other 2 days of the week, such as going for walks. You should try to enjoy yourself and have fun doing it, not to feel that you're in a militaristic boot-camp. Have fun whilst exercising, then you're more likely to build this into your daily routine.

You may be wondering why you should bother? Well the answer is simple: this is the only body you have, you need to look after it, you deserve to be as healthy as you can be, and the results from moving that little bit more each day will build up, and you'll notice a massive change in your overall health.

If you're overweight, there are little day-to-day things that you may have noticed about your level of health in comparison to those who are not so overweight: If you try walking and talking with a fitter colleague across a building to another location, they can walk more quickly than you can, and you're quite out-of-breath, you may feel embarrassed that you're struggling to keep up with them, even more so, if they're older than you are. If you're out and about and a friend or family member calls you on the mobile, trying to talk and walk to them, puts you really out of breath, because you're unfit walking and talking is difficult. If you have to run anywhere, to chase after a child/dog, or to catch a train or bus for example, you're wheezing and red faced by the time you get there and it takes a long time for you to catch your breath afterwards. When you go into shop, you find it hard to find clothes in your size, and if they do have your size, in comparison to the much smaller sizes, the cloths hang like shapeless sacks. You may notice on public transport, that instead of just fitting into one seat, your body is actually taking up one and a half seats, meaning that if someone sits next to you, you're really squashed and uncomfortable. You'll notice that you have rolls of fat on your body and wobbles where you shouldn't have. You'll sweat more in hot weather because you're carrying more weight around. Your thighs may rub together at the top if you're wearing a skirt or dress.

None of this is coming at it from a fat-shaming perspective. Being overweight doesn't make you a bad person. You're still you! The wonderful person with all your incredible qualities, skills and abilities that you have. But, in truth you're not as healthy as you could be, and you're putting yourself at risk of many illnesses the longer this goes on: such as heart attacks, Type II Diabetes, Cancer and strokes; in fact being overweight increases your risk of getting these by double!!!!! If you diet and exercise you can add at least a third longer onto your life.

When you exercise more, this not only has good things that happen to you physically, but mentally too. Exercising can boost your self-esteem and confidence, it can help you to get a good night's sleep, it can put you in a good mood, give you more energy, reduce your feelings of stress, reduce the chances of you feeling depressed, and reduce the risk of later in life, you getting Dementia or Azheimer's disease.

Physically exercising will make your bones and joints stronger and healthier. Your immune system will get a great boost, making you less prone to catching cold/flu viruses and any other bugs. Exercising will improve your shape, when you consistently exercise you will see that your muscles become more defined and take on a pleasant shape, and the fat on your body will disappear as you tone up. Your posture will become better. Exercise as mentioned releases endorphins into your body, which are known as 'happy hormones' and will make you feel wonderfully positive. By exercising you'll keep any weight that you've lost off!

You don't have to sign up to a gym, join any sports clubs, or even commit to great stretches of time. If you're fairly new to exercise currently, this book just wants you to find small pockets of time, 5 minutes can be a good start, and move more within that time. This book just wants you to move more, in a way that you enjoy; so that you can build up to doing more of it. Don't do something that makes you unhappy or else you aren't going to stick to this.

There WILL be some 'movement' that you enjoy, and this could take many many forms. It could be a certain type of exercise; it could be more dance oriented exercise such as Zumba; it could just be dance, ie putting on some music you love and dancing round your front room like a maniac to it, it's all exercise, it all counts. It could be roller-blading; ice-skating; rock-climbing; swimming; skiing; gardening; walking swiftly; trampolining; ten-pin bowling; playing on Wii Fit; jogging etc. If you like walking or jogging, you could get a FitBit or even just a pedometer, to measure how many steps you have taken. Or you could use a phone app, such as something like 'Map My Run' to measure the distance of the route you have walked or run. If you're using an app that does measure your route you can make it even more fun by trying to walk/jog a route that draws a picture, or spells out a name. Whatever exercise you do, should leave you feeling better than you did before.

It's important to start exercising at a time that suits you, whether that's today, tomorrow or next week. But, the sooner you start, the sooner you'll see good habits forming and excellent results for your body and mind. Don't overdo the exercise the first time you start, start with something small and achievable, and build upon this a little as time goes by. You don't have to increase things massively each day. It'd be better for you to do a small manageable amount of exercise every day, than one huge amount that puts you off, so you don't exercise again for weeks!

Do be realistic with your expectations about exercise. You're not going to look like a top performing athlete with defined muscles and a six-pack over night, but with time you'll get there. Look at exercise as a pleasant diversion away from the stresses of every-day life, it's a bit of time for you to take some 'time-out' and relax. Becoming toned, will follow with time, honestly!

So, when you've reached the point of deciding you are going to exercise, think about how much exercise you can commit to per week. Could you do up to 30 minutes per week? If so, what you could do is break down this time further. You could decide to do three lots of 10 minutes of exercise per week. Or if you don't want to start that high, you could do 6 lots of 5 minutes of exercise per week. EVERYBODY has at least 5 minutes out of their day where they can exercise. It's achievable and manageable. If you genuinely don't think you have 5 minutes out a day ... well then set your alarm clock 5 minutes earlier to get up and do the exercise first thing then. You're not going to miss out on 5 minutes extra of sleep ... but that would get your exercise quota in and done for the week. You need to also try to reduce the time that you spend sitting, by 15 minutes.

After a while of doing 30 minutes of exercise per week, you could up this to 90 minutes per week. This could be 3 lots of 30 minutes of exercise; or 6 lots of 15 minutes of exercise. What you could also be working on, is reducing the amount of time that you spend sitting per day. If you work in a very sedentary job, the last thing you want to be doing, is sitting solidly when you get home from work. If you can try to reduce the amount of time you spend sitting per day, by 15 minutes, this will be a big improvement in getting you moving more over the week, month and year! If you started at the stage one of doing 30 minutes of exercise per week, and reduced the time you spent sitting per day by 15 mins. This is a further 15 minutes on top of that.

If you've managed a month of doing 90 minutes of exercise per week, then you could move up to 150 minutes of exercise per week. This could be five lots of 30 minutes of exercise per week, or you could break it down into 10 lots of 15 minutes of exercise per week. If you've worked your way through the stages, and have reduced your sitting time by 15 minutes in stage 1, and a further 15 minutes in stage 2, then in this stage you need to again reduce the amount of time you spend sitting in a day, by a further 15 minutes. If you work in a sedentary role, there are easy ways of doing this. Instead of sitting through your morning or afternoon break, go for a walk during this time. If it's horrible weather outside, then simply walk around the building. You could also, if you catch public transport to work (or drive) get off the bus or tram stop one stop early to make yourself walk that little bit further. Or if you drive park further away so that you have that little bit more of a walk to get there. Get out for a walk in the early mornings or light summer nights after work. Instead of just slumping on the settee and watching TV, get out in your garden pulling up some weeds and watering plants for 15 minutes a day, as well as keeping you active and moving, your garden will benefit and look better for it too. If it's possible for you to walk to a local shop rather than drive, then do so. We become too reliant upon our cars.

If you get into the habit of exercising more, this does mean that you could introduce a few more carbohydrates into your Ketogenic diet. Don't go overboard with these, and certainly don't do too many to start off with. Over time, you'll learn what is the right amount for you.

It is important to try and sit less, we've mentioned earlier in this chapter, about trying to sit 15 minutes less per day in the various stages of moving. If you watch a lot of TV, every time there's an advert make sure that you get up, and walk about, stretch and are active during that time. Stand and wash up, rather than using a dish-washer. Use a watering can to water the garden, rather than a hose, as this will mean more bending, stretching and walking about. Try looking at Facebook standing up, rather than sitting down. There will be things you can do standing, rather than just sitting. At work, move the bin so that you have to get up to put stuff in, rather than it being directly under your desk. Stand up when you're on the phone, great people from history such as Winston Churchill and Leonardo da Vinci used to have stand up desks. Do stretches at your desk. Walk to see colleagues in person, rather than sending an email, it's a great way to build up professional relationships as well as making you healthier.

There are little changes you can make, such as parking further away from the supermarket entrance, meaning you have to walk further. Always take the stairs and not elevators or lifts. Doing little changes like this will add up over the weeks. If you used to love doing something as a child, then do it again now as an adult and have as much fun. Go cycling, there are also park runs that you can join, and on some of them they have an inflatable obstacle course, foam, or a colour paint dash. Enjoy yourself as much as you can in being active.

You don't need expensive gym equipment or gym membership in order to lose weight, you can lose weight on a budget too. You can do push ups against a wall of your house, you can use baked-bean or soup cans as hand-weights to do bicep curls. You can use the back of a settee in order to plank. You can do jumping jacks on the spot. You can do a wall sit, where you stand with your back flat against a wall, walk your feet 2 feet in front of you, spread them about 6" apart, slide your back down the wall, bend your knees until they're at a 90 degree angle as though you are sitting in an invisible chair. All of these exercises you can do for just one minute at a time, which everyone can make the time for, and they will build your core strength. If you're a mum or dad with a small child in a push-chair, there are various exercises you can do as you push them for a walk including picking up your walking pace, squatting, doing different speed intervals for 30 seconds at a time, and a side stretch, and pendulum legs. You can do a wealth of exercises too when doing house-work such as tricep dips, calf raises, a straight arm raise with a broom or feather duster, leg lunges as you're vacuuming, and a squat whilst you're putting dishes in the dish-washer. You can do a work out when you're getting out of bed, a stretch, a side twist, knees up, a torso twist, and a power walk on the spot. There is no excuse to get exercise implemented into your routine.

Going for walks is a great way to get you moving and to improve your health. Walking will clear your head of all the things that go on throughout the day and clutter up your brain and make your head fuzzy. The fresh air as you walk seems to blow these all away and make all problems and issues become minor and more manageable. Walking is an excellent way to improve hear-health and it's also good for your wallet too, as it doesn't cost anything! There's no special equipment you need to purchase, just some comfortable shoes! You should ideally aim to be walking for 30 minutes 5 days a week. You don't have to do a 30 minute walk all in one go, you could break that into 3 ten minute walks. It has been shown that people who measure their steps with a pedometer, tend to do 2,000 more steps a day, than people who don't. It's best to briskly walk (because then you're working at a moderately intense level) , but even leisurely walking is good for you, so just get out there and do it. You're able to tell when you're walking briskly, because your heart will beat faster than normal and your breathing will be deeper than normal, and you're still able to carry on a conversation. You should feel a lovely warm glow. Your heart shouldn't be racing, and your breathing should still be regular. Wear comfortable shoes or trainers. If you can only walk briskly for a few minutes, that's fine, build up the amount of minutes you can do over time. Always ensure that you start off your walk slowly, and end slowly, this will act as a warm-up and cool-down for you and prevent any muscle injuries.

Once you get it into you mind that you want to move more, you'll see opportunities to do so, all around you in day-to-day life.

Positivity

This section of the book is titled 'Positivity' this is because on the Ketogenic diet, we're aware it's more than just a 'diet' it encompasses a whole lifestyle change. We want to take a holistic approach, which includes the whole of you as a person. We want to take into account your feelings, your happiness, your self-confidence, and striving to be the best person that you can be. We want you to have more energy, be less stressed, move and exercise more in fun ways. Doesn't this sound great? Doesn't this sound caring? Who doesn't want to smile more, be happier, have more energy, more confidence, achieve more of your goals and aims?

By having the right frame of mind, having positive thoughts, loving yourself, having an awareness of your own will power and determination are central to transforming your body through diet and exercise this will help your Ketogenic lifestyle be much more successful. By choosing to do this mentally, you're making a commitment. The fact that you've decided you want to engage with a Ketogenic diet is a brilliant step in the right direction to transform your life for the better! Well done you! You also definitely have the strength and ability to do this and be successful, you just need to unlock your own superpowers in your mind, and start strongly believing in yourself. Every positive thing you do is a step towards a healthier future for you.

You can start off by setting a realistic goal weight that you want to achieve. You can write that down, but now set a mini-goal to strive towards that will keep you motivated, for example, losing 5% of your body weight can be an excellent starting point. Once you achieve your first mini-goal you deserve to do a victory dance and celebrate.

There are other ways that you can measure success on a Ketogenic diet, it doesn't just have to be by pounds lost on the scales. You could measure the inches that you've lost from parts of your body, your upper arms, tummy, hips, bum, and thighs. You could either do this with a tape-measure, or simply by noticing when you need to tighten your belt buckle, or when clothes that did feel tight feel comfortable, or even loose! You can notice things like your healthy generally improving and you becoming much fitter, ie. Not being so out of breath when you walk up the stairs, or you generally have more energy in the evenings after work. Congratulate yourself for making healthier food choices, avoiding carbohydrates, and incorporating more good fats into your diet, that will change your metabolism for the better and burn the fat, and help you lose weight; keeping your blood sugar and insulin levels low. Every day make a note of how you feel in a notebook, on a table you create or online with a tracker, and hopefully you'll see a pattern of more positivity appearing.

Remind yourself every day about how important you are, and that you deserve the best, and to be happy. Often in life we can place other people as a higher priority before ourselves, whether that's our children, partner or parents, but their ow health and wellbeing can suffer. You are as important as them, and as deserving to take time to make yourself healthy food, and have time for exercise. You do need to take care of yourself, in order to be able to help others.

Keep thinking positively. Be kind about yourself, and don't put yourself down. If you look in the mirror and see parts of yourself that you're not so keen on; instead praise all the bits you do like. Whether that's the colour of your eyes, your hair, your freckles, dimples, nice hands, pretty coloured nails etc. Also remember there's a lot more to a person other than their appearance, whether that's their personality, their kindness, their ability to do things, their sense of humour, intelligence etc. Be kind to yourself. Think now about 10 things that you like about yourself, big or small. This could be what a great parent, sister, brother, daughter, husband etc you are. You could be a great friend. You could be good with animals. There might be a part of your body you do love. There could be a particular meal that is a signature dish that you make very well. You may have a great sense of humour and be able to make others laugh and smile. You may like your toes, or ankles, or fingers. You may be a great gardener and grow the best flowers, or vegetables around. You may have great spatial awareness. You could be the person who is great at reading a map, or finding their way to places on a journey. You may be great at maths and be able to participate in the maths challenge on Countdown. You may have a great memory for general knowledge and be great at pub quizzes. There will always be things that are unique and special about you and worthy of merit, things about you that are pretty cool. Any time a negative thought about yourself creeps into your head, then replace that with a positive thought about one of the many things that you like about yourself, or you're good at. If anyone compliments you, don't even in a jokey way turn that into a put-down, instead just say 'thank you.' Once you have belief in yourself, others will pick up on your positive energy.

You do need to put yourself first some of the time, and take time to do what makes you happy, whether that's reading, embroidery, going for walks, painting, a long uninterrupted soak in the bath; a treatment day at a spa; going paintballing or on a

Segway; meeting up with friends at a pub etc. If you constantly put other's needs before yourself, you'll become bitter and will 'snap' at some point, and become unhappy because you're pleasing everyone else but you. This isn't being selfish, everyone deserves some time to do what makes them happy. This is about creating balance to your life. When you're stressed, snappy and irritable, this will have you reaching for sugary sweet snacks and carbohydrates, that you'll get your endorphins from, rather than life. But, unfortunately when you do this, you're not sticking to your Ketogenic diet, you'll come out of Ketosis or prevent yourself from reaching, and you'll not be eating food that is good for you.

Things you can do to relax can include taking a nap, which can often be a good way to sort thoughts out in a really busy head. You'll find that when you wake up, you're less tired and more able to think easily and make better decisions. You could just decide to sit somewhere that is comfy and quiet for a few minutes, and concentrate on breathing slowly in and out. You could take a book to read if you want a bit of escapism from daily-life. You could decide to have a soak in the bath, and add either some Epsom salts, or nice flavoured bubble bath to soak away any achey muscles and joints, which will help you have a good night's sleep. Listening to music can be an excellent way to relax and put you into a calm mindset. If there are songs that especially cheer you up, and have an upbeat feel that make you want to dance, then play them. Stretching can be a great way to relieve tension from your body. There is also an app called 'Headspace' which can help you to learn Mindfulness techniques that can boost your mood and make you feel more positive, and can help you to become more resilient with what life throws at you.

Adding some creativity into your life can help you to unwind and relax. There are many things you can do, that will help you to be more creative. You could decide to draw something, paint something, write a song or a poem, play an instrument, create something out of wool by knitting or crocheting, get an adult colouring book. You could decide to set up a Pinterest account and make some boards that interest you. You could take up photography. You may decide to make some clothes, try tye-dye, make something for the house.

If you want to ensure you have more happiness in your life, there are simple things that can achieve that. Go for a ten-minute walk, and appreciate all the nature around you. You don't have to live in the countryside to do this. Look at the sky, the colours, the clouds, the birds in it. Find some flowers or beautiful trees or plants, look at their shape, colour and texture. Laugh out loud, find some jokes on the Internet that appeal to your sense of humour, or some funny memes, or watch a YouTube clip of your favourite comedian. Make a 'happy playlist' of all your favourite upbeat tunes that you love. Do practice being grateful and appreciative for all the little things in life, it makes us kinder and happier, and you'll find that the more you're grateful and appreciative of, the more good things will come to you in life. Do remember also to try and get a good night's sleep. When you're sleep deprived you feel constantly exhausted, irritable, snappy, and everything feels a chore. Write down at least three things that you're grateful for; do look back at your list whenever you're feeling down as a reminder of the good things in your life. Do remember to give compliments to others, because by doing this, you'll cheer them up and you'll get back what you give, and who doesn't want more compliments in their life. Try to give genuinely meant compliments though, not just compliments for compliments sake. This could be if someone is looking nice, or if someone has made you a particularly nice cup of tea, if someone has performed a job well etc.

It's been proved that if you have someone who can support you with your new healthy lifestyle you're much more likely to succeed at it. Don't worry if you are on your own, this doesn't mean you won't have success, because you will get support from your weekly group, and leader. However, you could encourage another person to participate in activities with you, or you could enlist the support of a good friend, a husband, wife, or other relative. If you wander off track with your diet/healthy eating plan, then these people are all here to support you and get you back on track. Everyone is human, and occasionally things may slip and not go to plan, these people will give you a hug and help you through the tough times.

Many people who start on a Ketogenic diet, have dieted before, and that diet hasn't necessarily been as successful as you'd like it to be, or it's case of it worked, but the weight has crept back on. That's the past, that's history, don't dwell on what has happened in the past. Any time you decide to start on a diet, this is your new future, you can make this diet work for you. This is the only time that matters right now. How you've behaved in the past, does not matter, your future can be as you choose it to be. Have faith in yourself that you can achieve it. Cheer yourself on, give yourself a positive talking to. Pat yourself on the back for any accomplishments you achieve. Stop thinking that you're not capable, or can't do it. You can. It can be difficult adjusting to a diet and what you can and can't eat, but it is truly worth it.

You need to learn that eating carbohydrate food won't make you feel any better. If you've had a rubbish day, and you reach for biscuits or chocolate, it won't make you feel better. By eating it, you'll only add the feeling of guilt of eating naughty food, and feel a bit like you've failed at part of your diet. If you ever do this, and most of us will on a diet, then don't dwell on it, and just move on and tomorrow is a brand-new day. If you feel angry, lonely, sad, anxious, bored or miserable, you may think that food is the answer, but it's honestly not. It's much better to work out what is really going on, and to find a way to deal with it.

If you're stressed, instead of snacking on naughty food, try listening to three minutes of happy upbeat music. Write a list of the things you have to do, as this will lend structure to what you have to do, and make it seem more manageable and easier to deal with. Writing lists are a great way of getting everything that is cluttering up your head and trying to be remembered, out of your head and onto paper. By putting it on paper, you no longer have to stress and worry about the things you have to do, as it's all there in black and white in front of you, ready to be crossed off the list once you've completed it.

If you're eating because you're bored, then do something to liven up your life. You could decide to do something that you've not done in ages, whether this is visiting a local tourist attraction, do a jigsaw, a Sudoku puzzle, write a letter to a friend or family member, fly a kite etc.

If you're eating because you're lonely, then making connections with people is much better than eating food. Phone a friend for a chat, join a club, join a book club, volunteer at a charity shop, or working with animals or people. Spend an hour on social media, using Facebook or Twitter is a great way to connect with others. Often places near where you live will have 'Meet Up' groups. Meetup is great for finding people who are like-minded and enjoy doing the same things as you. This IS NOT a dating site, it is simply a site to find friends who like the same activities. It could be a writer's group; it could be a group of people who like to visit the cinema to see new films. It could be people who like going for walks (rambling); other people like going to see live gigs, others enjoy meals out, theatre trips, discussing history or philosophy etc.

There are things that will happen as part of life, for example family parties with birthday cake, nights out, popcorn at the cinema, fish and chips on the beach and so on. This is part of life, it is important to enjoy these from time to time; just not ALL the time. As a treat these are perfectly fine, you're human and it's expected. It's about trying to live a well-balanced life, and if 80 – 90% of your food choices can be healthy ones, that's a good balance. Don't try to be perfect, as no-one can be all the time. If you have a naughty treat, keep this in perspective against ALL the healthy food you've eaten that week, and don't beat yourself up for having it; don't guilt trip yourself over it. Simply move on and start being healthy again at the next opportunity.

Also, be REALLY careful, not to think, 'Oh, I've ruined my diet now' by having one small naughty treat, and using that as an excuse to carry on eating everything naughty and just give up all together. It was one naughty thing, get over it, get back on track, just ensure your next meal and the ones after are healthy.

Do remember that there are lots of ways you can judge how well you're doing on a diet, it's not all just about what you weigh on the scales. You may find that jewellery you wear become looser. You may find parts of your body such as your collar bone or hip bone become more prominent once you start to lose weight. You may find that you have more energy to run around playing with younger family members. You may find out from tests at the GP that your blood pressure and cholesterol levels have lowered or become within normal range. You may start to feel much more comfortable when having photos taken, or when going clothes shopping.

Eating Out

When you eat out make your best guestimate for what the food your eating is worth in terms of fat, protein and carbohydrates from the food that you would normally eat at home. Note it down, enjoy your meal and don't dwell any more on the carbs. Don't let worrying about the carbohydrate content detract from your meal.

Try to make sensible choices with the food you have whilst you're out. You know that foods rich in fresh grass-fed meat and fresh-fish, oil, cream, butter and cheese are going to better on a Ketogenic diet. You know that green vegetables will be appropriate low-carbohydrate accompaniment.

With many eating places, you are able to look at the menu before you go out, to work out what are the best options for you. If you decide before you go out, you'll be less likely to change your mind, or be swayed by other people's orders when you get there. If you know in advance that you'll be eating out, you could ensure that the other things you eat that day are quite low in carbohydrates.

Soup for starter can be a nice way to fill up, so that you're not as hungry throughout the main or dessert. Clear broth based soups and vegetable soups are probably likely to be lower and contain more sodium which is good for you on a ketogenic diet.

Do remember to drink lots of water when you're eating out, you can see the chapter above on how water helps for weight loss. It will fill you up and ensure that you're really hungry, it will also help to aid digestion. Chew your food slowly, remember to talk to the people you're there with, and not simply have your head down eating food quickly. Do remember to still track what you've eaten when you're out.

If you've over-indulged when you've gone for a night out for a meal, and have gone over your daily 5% carbohydrates, then don't dwell on it. It will happen sometimes. Simply just move on, and ensure that your next meals are healthy and within your carbohydrate

For some cuisines, certain sauces can be quite high in sugar. It has been worked out that Sweet n' Sour sauce from many Chinese restaurants can contain between 13 – 31 teaspoons of sugar. At a pub, try to pick grilled salmon, chicken dishes, or a fillet steak. There are so many coffee shops that have opened up, again it would be impossible to list them all, and all the types of coffee in one book, you could consider asking them to make your coffee with almond or coconut milk in order to make this better for you. In order to make you coffee less high carbohydrate, you could decide to have sweetener rather than sugar (ideally something natural live Stevia). An Americano doesn't contain any milk, it's an expresso diluted with water. A frappe will often have sugar or syrup in it. It a coffee has 'whip' listed on its title, it is likely to contain whipped cream and this is a good option on a Ketogenic diet. If you decide to eat at fast food places, there are better choices that you can make at McDonalds or Burger King. At McDonalds and Burger King, you can ask for burgers without the bun.

It is a proven fact that when we 'watch' and track what we eat, this helps us to lose weight, because when you keep track of what you eat, you become MUCH more aware of what you're putting into your body. All the little snacks that seem innocuous, all the desserts, all the drinks, how much bread you're eating per day, how many sweets, packets of crisps, takeaways, are suddenly there in black and white, and there's no denying that you've eaten them, and all of a sudden you can easily see where all the calories, and thus all the weight has crept up from. Without tracking our food, we do definitely eat more than we should and more unhealthy food. It is important to check that you're not consuming more carbohydrates than you should.

By tracking your carbohydrate intake, you will be MUCH more likely to stick to your 5% carbohydrate allowance that has been allocated to you. The Ketogenic diet isn't intended to make your life difficult, or complicated, or needlessly time-consuming, so whilst you need to track your food, this doesn't need to overtake your life or be done to the nth degree; often giving your best estimate can be good enough. If you feel you simply don't have time to calculate carbohydrates one day, you could write down a rough idea of what you've eaten; or you could even take some photos with your phone, and calculate the next day. You could use an online tracker, a notebook, or create a table. In your notebook or online tracker, you could use emoticons that show if you're very unhappy, unhappy, neutral, happy, or very happy. You could document how many hours sleep you've had the night before (again a Fitbit would tell you this). You could note in your notebook or journal what the best bits of your week have been, or the worst bits of your week, foodie faves this week, and overall how your week was, the week's weight change and your challenge for the following week. You can access online trackers on your computer or laptop; or if you prefer to work more on the go, your can get mobile apps to track food/drink/water/exercise.

Once you've eaten a meal. It can take 20 minutes for your stomach to send a message to your brain that you're full. So, before going back for seconds, give your stomach time to notify your brain that you've actually had enough to eat.

Hopefully you'll find that with a Ketogenic diet, you'll no longer have food cravings, because the food is good and healthy, and you'll see it not as a 'diet' but a way of life that is manageable and works for you.

Just because you're eating out, doesn't mean that you HAVE to follow the usual norms. Whilst many restaurants will encourage you to have a starter, a main and a dessert. You don't have to. The choice is yours. You could decide to have the start and main, but not dessert. Or, the main and dessert, but not starter. Do have a plan of what you'll eat before you go. Try not to arrive at the restaurant ravenously hungry as you won't make the best diet decisions in that state. If you're able to, order first, so that other people's food choices don't influence you.

The size of portions you eat when you eat out, again can make quite a big difference to your diet. There are things you can eat at home, that would give you a much healthier alternative to some foods you get when you eat out. For example 'cauliflower rice' can be used instead of Indian, Chinese or Thai style rice, so it's MUCH lower in Carbohydrates. You grate or blend a cauliflower so it's a similar size to rice, and add the spices of your choosing. You can make fish and chips at home, and perhaps have just a few sweet potato chips as a low-carb treat. You can make a low-carbohydrate pizza which looks delicious and this has a mozzarella cheese base and doesn't use any flour at all.

Alcohol

When you're eating out, or perhaps even just socialising with friends, it's worth noting that drinkin alcohol can take you out of the state of Ketosis. If you want to drink alcohol, it's best to opt for a dry wine, rather than a sweet wine.

Planning

When you're on a diet, many people feel a little like Jekyll and Hyde, where they desperately want to lose weight, but then they have this naughty character inside, that says: 'go on, treat yourself, eat that whole box of chocolates or some slices of toast, or a bowl of cereal or rice,' it's a constant battle between good and evil. You 'may' be a person with excellent will power and you may naturally be able to work out your carbohydrate intake on the go throughout the day. But, many people, especially when they're first starting out on the diet, find this hard to do, and if you're not careful you can end up eating too many of carbohydrates early in the day, and not having enough left for the rest of the evening. Which can result in either you going over your carbohydrate allowance and coming out of or not maintaining ketosis, or being hungry one evening.

If you plan your carbohydrates out prior to the start of the day, you'll automatically know what you're having for all your meals, and snacks, and there's no nasty surprises of ruining your chances of ketosis. It also makes it MUCH less likely that you'll reach for food that hasn't been accounted for, by a hasty rash decision, where you've grabbed food out of hunger.

If you want to, you could plan-out a whole week's worth of meals (see Chapter 3). Or, if this seems too much to do at once, then just plan on a day by day level.

You don't actually need any special tracker sheets, in order to monitor what you eat. A simple piece of paper split into 3 columns for Breakfast, Lunch and Dinner/Tea, and 7 rows for each day of the week works just as effectively.

There will be some parts of your daily diet that are predictable, for example if you need cream for cups of coffee, broth for a salty drink, pink Himalayan rock salt etc.

Conclusion

I hope that by the end of reading this book: *Ketogenic Diet*, that you'll see that this is true, and that a Ketogenic is available to anyone and everyone. It's very affordable, it's good wholesome food, it's nothing complicated, you don't require any specialist equipment, there's nothing faddy about the diet; instead it's straightforward common sense, of cutting out carbohydrates and eating more fat. Some people are under the impression that meat is expensive and that they simply can't afford to eat it very often, and therefore think that a ketogenic/low-carbohydrate diet wouldn't be accessible to them. We're not however talking about expensive joints of meat that you need to purchase. Many of the recipes include chicken, bacon, turkey, ham, minced beef, all of which you can pick up inexpensively, and because these are the core bits to your diet, and you're no longer purchasing processed foods or carbohydrates, you will see no difference to the cost of your shopping bills.

This diet is perfect if you're wanting to lose weight and improve your health. This book has explained all about a ketogenic diet and the balance of food, and the types of food you need to eat, in order to achieve the state of ketosis. It also mentions the types of food that you should avoid. By eating a

Ketogenic diet, there are so many benefits for your health too. Not only will you lose weight, but your cholesterol will improve, your blood sugar and blood pressure will reduce, and there's a wealth of other conditions/diseases that by eating a Ketogenic diet, you're at less risk of contracting.

This book has hopefully shown you that you don't need to eat less; you just learn to eat smarter food options, much less carbohydrates (only about 5%) and much greater fats (about 75%). You'll have learned the sensible rate that you should ideally be losing weight at. You'll have learned about the foods that you can, and can't eat (it's mostly just carbohydrates that are the key restriction). There are foods however, that are more sensible options, that will make you feel fuller for longer. You'll have learned how the Body Mass Index (BMI) is calculated, and how you work out approximately where your BMI is, but also to take into account that this isn't set in stone, just an approximate guide. By losing 10% of your body weight, this can have a dramatic positive impact. Chapter 15 will give you lots of information about Super Foods, and you can pick as many of these as possible to include in your daily meals for good results. You'll learn about the benefits of tracking food, and the general principles behind Ketogenic diets and an ethos of truly wanting you to lose weight, and keep the weight off permanently. You'll learn about planning your meals for best effect.

I hope you've enjoyed reading this, and good look on achieving and maintaining Ketosis.

CPSIA information can be obtained
at www.ICGtesting.com
Printed in the USA
LVOW10s0634191217
560231LV00022B/1200/P